DRUG NAMES DECODED,

3rd Edition

By Tony Guerra, Pharm.D.

Drug Names Decoded, 3rd Edition

Copyright © 2013 by Tony Guerra, Pharm.D.

ISBN: 978-1-304-60757-7

To Mindy,

Brielle, Rianne, and Teagan

FOREWORD

My pharmacology students struggled with the correct pronunciation and memorization of drug names. Because I had been pronouncing them for so long, I didn't realize I had "learned the language" and I couldn't see how to best help students get around the challenge. I took a week to try to learn French, a language I didn't know. Immediately, I understood the three major challenges:

1. It's tough to learn and memorize a word if you can't pronounce it. Most French words use the same Roman "A to Z" alphabet as English, but the pronunciations are very different or unfamiliar just like generic drug names.

2. In the pharmacology textbooks I used, I found many generic names in the first chapters. Those generic names are in the language of organic and biochemistry, a class that most of my students had not taken. In contrast, the language books always define a word immediately before or after introducing it so nothing is unfamiliar.

3. Finally, I found clues in the brand names of the drugs that hinted what they were for, as I found French words that had remnants of English words (cognates and false-cognates) that I already knew.

After opening myself up to language as a key to learning pharmacology, I moved from the pursuit of learning French to learning Latin. Latin has a myriad of suffixes and strange endings and cannot be readily translated word for word. I now felt like a student again: frustrated, lost and pounding my head asking myself, "Why don't I get this?" In addition, my triplet daughters were born taking away a significant amount of my time. I could only learn in small, often interrupted bites.

Eventually, I accepted two facts: 1. I needed to get help from other people to learn a new language efficiently. 2. These people, on YouTube at least, were writing fun mnemonics (memory devices) and songs. A song helped me learn the six endings for the present indicative of the verb "to love" in Latin :

Person/Number	English Verb	Latin Verb
I	Love	Amo
You	Love	Amas
He, She, It	Loves	Amat
We	Love	Amamus
You all	Love	Amatis
They	Love	Amant

Similar to pharmacology, the stem of the word love, ama-, stays the same similar to how the suffixes or prefixes often stay the same for pharmacologic drugs. After this realization I made up the *Cardiode to Joy* which goes to the beat of Beethoven's *Ode to Joy* which is found in the cardiology chapter of this book. Memorizing words alone will not get you there. It is with a combination of mnemonics, repetition and some fun that can make pharmacology a favorite subject.

TABLE OF CONTENTS

INTRODUCTION

Yuo cna raed tihs bceuase a preosn raeds a wolhe wrod nad nto jsut lteters. As lnog sa teh frist adn lsat lteters aer crrocet, it is lgebile.

You can read this because a person reads a whole word and not just letters. As long as the first and last letters are correct, it is legible.

Similarly, many drugs with similar spellings can be confused, just like identical twins or triplets. As you get to know their subtle differences, it becomes easy to tell them apart. Take the following quiz to see how much easier it is to tell two drugs apart that are spelled similarly, if you know a little bit about them.

1. **Use either Aricept or AcipHex.** *Which helps improves perception? Which affects the pH of acid?*

   _____is an Alzheimer's medication.
   _____is a proton pump inhibitor.

2. **Use either captopril or carvedilol.** *Drugs that end in –lol are beta blockers Drugs that end in –pril are ACE inhibitors.*

   _____is an ACE inhibitor.
   _____is a beta blocker.

3. **Use either Celexa or Celebrex.** *Which relaxes someone who is depressed? Which celebrates relief from pain?*

   _____ is a non-steroidal anti-inflammatory drug.
   _____ is an antidepressant.

4. **Use either Colace or Cozaar.** *Which doesn't make your colon race? Which affects the RAAS?*

   _____is a stool softener.
   _____is a blood pressure medication.

5. **Use either atorvastatin or nystatin.** *Some cholesterol drugs end in –vastatin. Myco- means fungus and the brand name for nystatin is Mycostatin.*

    _____ is a cholesterol-lowering medicine.
    _____ is an antifungal.

6. **Use either digoxin (Lanoxin) or Levothyroxine.** *Which comes from the digitalis plant? Which affects thyroid?*

    _____is for thyroid replacement.
    _____is to strengthen cardiac contraction.

7. **Use either Lopressor or Lyrica.** *Which makes you lyrical after becoming pain free? Which is to lower blood pressure?*

    _____ is a beta blocker for blood pressure.
    _____ is a medicine to relieve neuropathic pain.

8. **Use either Neurontin or Motrin.** *Which has the root of neuron? Which better rhymes with aspirin, a non-steroidal?*

    _____is a non-steroidal anti-inflammatory drug.
    _____is for neuropathic pain.

9. **Use either oxycodone or Oxycontin.** *Which has part of continuous in the name? Which has one in the name?*

    _____ is long acting oxycodone
    _____ is short acting oxycodone

10. **Use either Paxil or Plavix.** *Which vexes platelets? Which is the generic for the SSRI paroxetine?*

    _____is a blood thinner.
    _____is an antidepressant.

How did you do? Did you get at least one right in each question?

I bet you were close to 10 out of 10. This book will help you learn what to look for in a drug name, how to pronounce the drug properly, and teach you a mnemonic or memory tool to help you remember the drug.

Learning the drug names will flow easily because they are in a special order, an order in which the drug before it has something to do with the drug after. First, let's learn a little bit about where these drug names come from.

I. DRUG NAME ORIGINS

HOW IS A DRUG NAME FORMED?
With each drug, there are three types of names.

1) The chemical name

First, there is the most complex name, the IUPAC (International Union of Pure and Applied Chemistry) standard name, which makes perfect sense to a chemist who might want to draw the molecule.

(RS)-2-(4-(2-methylpropyl)phenyl)propanoic acid.

Second, there is an older way a chemist named compounds—the common name.

Iso-**bu**tyl-**pro**panoic-**phen**olic acid which becomes I bu pro phen, **ibuprofen**, the generic name.

2) The generic name

While this transformation to ibuprofen is an improvement, it has four syllables. Drug companies prefer to use names that have two to three syllables.

3) The brand/trade name

Two brand names for ibuprofen include Advil and Motrin, both with two easy-to-pronounce syllables, but do not resemble ibuprofen are used as the brand name because they include *plosives* to make powerful memorable stops in the word. A strong word sounds like strong medicine.

Say each of the following letters and see if you can feel it in your tongue or nose.

Tongue blade occlusion: *t or d*

Tongue body occlusion: *k or g*

Lip occlusion: *b or p*

Nasal stops: *m or n*

Motrin has an m, a nasal stop; t, a tongue blade occlusion; and n, another nasal stop. This forces the person saying the word to stop their breath three times, slowing the pronunciation and keeping it on the tongue and/or nose longer, making it seem very strong.

CHEMICAL ORIGINS

Generic drug names often come from small pieces of the very long chemical names included in the drugs. Read these next terms out loud carefully working through the pronunciation of each. You will quickly see that some pronunciations are identical to what you would expect, but some are very different.

In organic chemistry the word "but" is pronounced "byoot", "fur" is pronounce "fyoor", and the word "one" is pronounced "own" because these are no longer individual words, but parts of bigger chemical names. Making mistakes and seeing the differences for yourself will help you remember the correct pronunciations, so don't feel bad about stumbling on a few.

ORGANIC CHEMISTRY WORD PARTS PRACTICE

These words indicate the number of carbon atoms in an attached molecule made up only of carbon and hydrogen:

Methyl – *Methyl*phenidate	"METH-ill"
Ethyl – Fentan*yl*	"ETH-ill"
Propyl – Meto*pro*lol	"PROP-ill"
Butyl – Al*but*erol	"BYOOT-ill"

Levo and dextro mean left and right respectively:

Levo - *Levo*thyroxine	"LEE-vo"
Dextro - *Dex*methylphenidate	"DEX-trow"

These words mean there is a specific element in each molecule:

Thio (sulfur) – Hydrochloro*thi*azide	"THIGH-oh"
Chloro (chlorine) – Hydro*chloro*thiazide	"KLOR-oh"
Hydro (hydrogen) – *Hydro*codone/APAP	"HIGH-droe"

These words are branches that attach to the central molecule:

Acetyl – Levetir*acet*am	"Uh-SEAT-ill"
Alcohol – Tramad*ol*	"AL-kuh-haul"
Amide – Loper*amide*	"UH-myde"
Amine – Diphenhydr*amine*	"UH-mean"
Disulfide – *Disulf*iram	"DIE-sulf-eyed"
Furan – *Fur*osemide	"FYOOR-an"
Guanidine – Cimet*idine*	"GWAN-eh-dean"
Hydroxide – Magnesium *Hydroxide*	"HI-drox-eyed"
Imidazole – Omepr*azole*	"im-id-AZ-ole"
Ketone – Spironolact*one*	"KEY-tone"
Phenol – Acetamino*phen*	"FEN-ole"
Sulfa – *Sulfa*methoxyzole	"SULL-fuh"

Some drugs are named:

- **By what they do for the patient, also called the therapeutic class:** Anti-depressant
- **By their chemical structure:** Tricyclic antidepressants (TCA) (three rings in the compound)
- **By the receptor they affect:** Beta-blockers
- **By the neurotransmitter they affect:** Selective serotonin reuptake inhibitor (SSRI)

You'll become familiar with these as we progress through the book.

II. PRONUNCIATION

WHERE IS THE STRESSED SYLLABLE?

Tony – My first name translates into two easy-to-pronounce one-syllable English words, toe and knee with the stress on the toe. The stressed syllable will be in all CAPS.

Guerra – Cannot be pronounced with spoken English. I tell people it's pronounced like Sara with a G, but in reality there is an *erre* sound of rolling r's that is not found in spoken English.

The most famous last name in pronunciation is Boiardi, but he, Ettore Boiardi, chose to put the phonetic "Boyardee" on his Italian food so it would be pronounced correctly. But with a quick lesson in poetry, you can make it easier for someone to pronounce your name.

Poetry used to be taught to help learn *rhetoric*, or improving a speaker's ability to perform. In pharmacology, it can be invaluable in helping students say the drug names better. There are symbols for poetic meter and we can use these to make this simple:

(U) = unaccented and the slash (/) = accented

The accented, unaccented form / U is called a **trochee**. Examples of trochees include **MO**-trin which works a lot like *aspirin.*

U/ is an **iamb** such as a-**LEVE**, the brand name for a drug that *alleviates* inflammation. The accent follows the unstressed syllable.

/ U U is a **dactyl** with three syllables, one accented; then two unaccented like **LIP**-i-tor, a drug to reduce *lipids.*

U / U is an **amphibrach** which has three syllables, two unaccented with a central accent like Lan–**OX**–in, which can make your heart as strong as an *ox.*

Knowing the actual name of the poetic meter (trochee, iamb, dactyl, amphibrach) is not as important as connecting one word to another that has to do with the drug's function: Motrin to aspirin, Aleve to alleviate, Lipitor to lipids and Lanoxin to ox. Now try it with your name.

I would tell a person my name is a combination of two trochees: **TOE**-Knee (Tony) **GWHERE**-uh (Guerra) where the accent is on the first syllable. My first name is a combination of a toe and a knee. My last name is a "G" pushed in front of the word "where" and "uh"

How would you make it easier for a person to pronounce your name? Can you break it into small words?

Write it here:

PRONUNCIATION MISTAKES
It is important that you take your time, sound out one to two sylla-bles at a time when you are first saying the word; otherwise you might make one of these common mistakes.

One common pronunciation mistake come from trying to force a four-syllable-word into a more comfortable three syllables.

Atenolol, "uh-TEN-uh-lawl," is cut to atenol "at-EN-all"

Simvastatin, "SIM-va-stat-in," is cut to simvastin "SIM-vas-tin"

Sometimes a letter (r to t) is replaced:

A gene<u>r</u>ic drug becomes a gene<u>t</u>ic drug.

Or a letter (n) is omitted to make a known word:

Oxyco<u>n</u>tin "ox-e-CON-tin" is cut to oxy*cotton* "ox-e-COT-tin"

Or a sound is changed:

Metoprolol "meh-TOE-pruh-lawl" becomes "Met-UH-pro-lawl"

These mispronunciations take your credibility away. The terms in this book are written in easy to digest small words, familiar sounds, and proper names. For example:

TYLENOL comes from the chemical name N-ace**tyl**-para-amino-ph**enol** (APAP).
"TIE-Len-all"

TIE is the accented syllable. The tie you would wear with a suit.
Len is short for Lenny
all is a synonym for everything.

ALL CAPS = accented syllable // **Len** = a capitalized proper name

20

III. Brand names vs. Generic Names

BRAND NAME: OFTEN GIVES CLUE TO FUNCTION

The **brand name**, two to three syllables, often created by a market-ing firm, will sometimes hint at the *function* of a drug, i.e. Lopressor creates *lo*wered blood *press*ure

The **brand name** is like a two- to three-syllable nickname that *hints* at the drug's function, but by law, may not make a claim. The names are very much like a nickname such as Betsy or Jack. But a non-native English speaker would have no idea that Betsy comes from Elizabeth or Jack comes from Jonathan.

GENERIC NAME: CAN HELP GROUP DRUGS BY CLASS

Lopressor's four syllable generic name, metoprolol, has an –olol suffix which hints at the *drug class*, i.e. drugs that end in –olol are beta-blockers.

Generic names are like foreign language last names like mine that have a part that is unpronounceable because the sounds that form them are regularly used by *organic chemists* and *biochemists* and the brand names are distant relations to them.

How would you know that **Tylenol** and acetaminophen are related as brand and generic name without seeing the actual full chemical name N-ace**tyl**-para-aminoph**enol**?

How could you know that the brand-name drug Lopressor, which **lo**wers blood **press**ure, is metoprolol or that beta-blockers, a type of cardiac medication, end in –olol?

By using mnemonics.

IV. Mnemonics

HOMOPHONES

In grade school you may have learned the word "homophone" which is a word that may be spelled differently, but sounds the same.

Some examples include the words "there" and "their," "two" and "too," and "hear" and "here."

To remember which meaning should be associated with the word, the teacher may have told you to look inside the word for a clue:

In the word "their" you find "heir," such as the person who will inherit something. Then you can associate that the word "their" has to do with the possessive of a group of people versus "there" which means "in that place."

In the word "two" you can turn the w sideways to make a 3, spelling "t3o" so you can remember that two has to do with a number. Also, too has two o's, and you can remember that it has too many o's.

In the word "hear" you can find the word "ear" and you can remember that this form means to listen versus "here" which means "in this place."

Those clues are called **mnemonic** devices, something to help your memory. These also work in the memorization of drugs.

MNEMONICS IN PHARMACOLOGY

Prilosec contains "Pr" which can be short for "proton" (H^+), the associated ion with something acidic.

Prilosec contains "lo" which can be short for "low."

Prilosec contains "sec" which can be short for "secretion."

Prilosec's mechanism of action is to inhibit proton pumps and reduce the acid in a person's stomach. By looking at the name of the drug we can see that "proton" "low" "secretion" also means a reduction in protons, helping us remember the meaning of the word.

In the same light **Protonix** can be broken down into "proton" and "nix." To nix is a verb meaning "no" so "proton" + "nix" means "protons" + "no" or "no protons."

22

A NOTE ABOUT THE BRAND NAME MNEMONICS:

I didn't call anyone at any brand name drug companies. I just looked at each drug name and used my experience as a teacher of patho-physiology, pharmacology, and organic and biochemistry and made up something that seemed to makes sense, but more importantly will help the student remember the drug's drug class or function. The FDA does not allow a drug company to name a drug after its intend-ed use.

V. LEARNING THE COMPREHENSIVE DRUG LIST

Your next step is to learn each of the next 175 drugs (aspirin is used twice). I have created this order because drugs next to each other are related and those within a group are in a larger family based on physiologic system. As you go through, you'll start to form connec-tions between the drug before and the drug after. We will take it in small bite size steps, but I think you will be impressed with yourself when you can name every single drug's use from memory.

Many students like to use 3 by 5 cards to help them memorize drugs, but I wouldn't make 175 cards, rather, I would use the groupings starting on page 100 to halve that amount of notecards.

3x5 card front:

cime<u>tidine</u>
rani<u>tidine</u>

3x5 card back:

Class: H_2 blockers (-tidine)

Tagamet the H_2 an**tag**onist ci**met**idine, an upset stomach, will assist.

Pepcid reduces **pep**tic a**cid**ity, reducing ulcer morbidity.

COMPREHENSIVE DRUG LIST

Chapter 1 - Gastrointestinal

Calcium carbonate	Magnesium hydroxide	Cimetidine
Famotidine	Esomeprazole	Omeprazole
Pantoprazole	Ondansetron	Promethazine
Bismuth subsalicylate	Loperamide	*Lomotil
Polyethylene glycol	Docusate	Mesalamine

Chapter 2 – Musculoskeletal

Aspirin (ASA)	Ibuprofen	Naproxen
Meloxicam	Celecoxib	Acetaminophen
Fentanyl	Morphine	Oxycodone
Oxycodone/APAP	Hydrocodone/APAP	APAP/Codeine
Tramadol	ASA/APAP/Caffeine	Sumatriptan
Etanercept	Methotrexate (MTX)	Alendronate
Ibandronate	Colchicine	Allopurinol
Febuxostat		

Chapter 3 – Respiratory

Diphenhydramine	Cetirizine	Loratadine
Guaifenesin/DM	Guaifenesin/codeine	Mometasone
Methyprednisolone	Prednisone	Albuterol
Budesonide/Formoterol	Fluticasone/Salmeterol	Tiotropium
Montelukast	Pseudoephedrine	Epinephrine

Chapter 4 - Immune

Amoxicillin	Amox/Clavulanate	Cephalexin
Ceftriaxone	Cefepime	Erythromycin
Clarithromycin	Azithromycin	Ciprofloxacin
Levofloxacin	Doxycycline	Tetracycline
Amikacin	Gentamicin	Clindamycin
Metronidazole	SMZ/TMP	Vancomycin
Ethambutol	Isoniazid	Pyrazinamide
Rifampin	Amphotericin B	Fluconazole
Nystatin	Oseltamivir	Zanamavir
Acyclovir	Valacyclovir	Zidovudine

Chapter 5 - Neuro

Eszopiclone	Ramelton	Trazodone
Zolpidem	Citalopram	Escitalopram
Fluoxetine	Paroxetine	Sertraline
Venlafaxine	Amitriptyline	Isocarboxazid
Phenelzine	Tranylcypromine	Alprazolam
Clonazepam	Diazepam	Lorazepam
Dexmethylphenidate	Methylphenidate	Atomoxetine
Lithium	Chlorpromazine	Haloperidol
Olanzapine	Quetiapine	Risperidone
Carbamazepine	Divalproex	Phenytoin
Gabapentin	Pregabalin	Donepezil
Memantine	Levodopa/carbidopa	Selegeline
Meclizine	Scopolamine	Carisoprodol
Cyclobenzaprine	Benzocaine	Lidocaine

Chapter 6 - Cardiology

Mannitol	Furosemide	Hydrochlorothiazide
Triamterene/HCTZ	Spironolactone	Doxazosin
Propranolol	Metoprolol	Carvedilol
Enalapril	Lisinopril	Losartan
Olmesartan	Valsartan	Nitroglycerin
Diltiazem	Verapamil	Amlodipine
Nifedipine	Atorvastatin	Rosuvastatin
Simvastatin	Fenofibrate	Niacin
Enoxaparin	Heparin	Warfarin
Aspirin	Clopidogrel	Digoxin

Chapter 7 Endocrine

Glipizide	Glyburide	Metformin
Rosiglitazone	Glucagon	Insulin R
Insulin glargine	Levothyroxine	Propylthiouracil

Chapter 8 Renal/Reproductive

Oxybutynin	Tolterodine	Bethanechol
Sildenafil	Tadalafil	Tamsulosin
Dutasteride	Finasteride	*NuvaRing
*OrthoEvra	*Loestrin 24 Fe	*Tri-Sprintec

CHAPTER 1 GASTROINTESTINAL

I. PEPTIC ULCER DISEASE

Peptic ulcer disease (PUD) translates loosely to an ulceration of the **peptic** (PEP-tick) or digestive tract. Acid is an aggressive factor in the stomach that, if reduced, may allow an ulcer to heal. An antibiotic may also be used to treat the *Helicobacter pylori*, a helicopter-like organism often found in the ulcer, but in this section we will only focus on three drug classes: The antacid, the H_2-blocker, and the proton pump inhibitor (PPI).

ANTACIDS

An **antacid** is anti-acid without the "i" and is usually composed of a chemical like calcium, magnesium, or aluminum. **Calcium carbonate** (**Tums**) can supplement calcium in someone's diet and reduce acidity.

Antacids can chelate (bind with) antibiotics like tetracycline (Sumycin) and ciprofloxacin (Cipro) and should not be taken together with them. **Magnesium hydroxide** (**Milk of Magnesia**) is also an antacid, but can be used for constipation, so a patient will want to be careful how much they take.

CALCIUM CARBONATE (Tums)
"CAL-see-um CAR-bow-Nate" (TUMS)
Tums helps calm your **tum**my, so you can eat food that's yummy.

MAGNESIUM HYDROXIDE (Milk of Magnesia)
"mag-KNEES-e-um high-DROCK-side" (MILK of mag-KNEE-shuh)
Magnesium + **a** helps your stomach's frets go away.

H2 BLOCKERS (-TIDINE)

An **H_2 blocker** (more formally, H_2 receptor antagonist) stands for histamine two (H_2) blocker. When someone says, "I need an antihistamine," she thinks of allergic symptoms like sneezing, runny nose, etc. Those allergy antihistamines have to do with histamine one (H_1) receptors and we'll cover those in the antihistamine section. Histamine two causes the formation of acid, so blocking it blocks the production of acid. You'll notice **cimetidine (Tagamet)** and **famotidine (Pepcid)** both end in –tidine. How do we choose? **Cimetidine** inhibits the metabolism (breakdown) of certain other drugs in the cytochrome P450 system which is important for metabolism in the liver and because of this, **famotidine** is often preferred.

CIME<u>TIDINE</u> (Tagamet)
"sigh-MET-uh-dean" (TAG-uh-met)
Tagamet the H_2 anta**g**onist ci**met**idine, an upset stomach, will assist.

FAMO<u>TIDINE</u> (Pepcid)
"Fa–MOE–ti–dean" (PEP-Sid)
Pepcid reduces **pep**tic **acid**ity, reducing ulcer morbidity.

PROTON PUMP INHIBITORS (-PRAZOLE)

A **proton pump inhibitor** (PPI) blocks a pump that introduces protons into the stomach, making it less acidic. PPIs can be combined with antibiotics to create a triple therapy for ulceration to kill *H. pylori*.

While **esomeprazole (Nexium)**, **omeprazole (Prilosec)**, and **pantoprazole (Protonix)** all have the same ending –prazole, notice the only thing that separates **omeprazole** and **esomeprazole** is an es-. Chemicals may have a mirror image. Instead of calling them right- and left-handed, we call them R and S from the Latin words *rectus* (right) and *sinister* (left).

Usually the S form is more active biologically. Putting an "s" in front of omeprazole makes someprazole which would be pronounced "some" "prazole". Instead, the "es" allows for a separation between the S- and the compound, as a chemist would pronounce it.

Pantoprazole (Protonix) is very similar, sometimes called a "me-too drug" and allows for different drug companies to compete and keep drug prices down.

ESOMEPRAZOLE (Nexium)
"es-oh-MEP-rah-zole" (NECKS-see-um)
Nexium makes your stomach fine in the **next** hour, so **yum** you can say, and be no longer dour.

OMEPRAZOLE (Prilosec)
"oh-MEP-rah-zole" (PRY-low-sec)
Prilosec creates a **low sec**retion of **pro**tons.

PANTOPRAZOLE (Protonix)
"pan-TOE-pruh-zole" (PRO-tawn-icks)
Protonix nixes protons so your stomach is fixed.

II. NAUSEA, DIARRHEA AND CONSTIPATION

When a toxin is present, vomiting is good. However, with cancer chemotherapy, we know the **nausea's** cause. We want to prevent it with a drug like **ondansetron (Zofran)** or **promethazine (Phenergan)** which has rectal dosage forms.

Diarrhea leads to dehydration and sometimes we need to intervene and use over-the-counter medications like **bismuth (Pepto-Bismol)** or **Imodium (Loperamide)**. But if a patient needs something stronger and by prescription, **diphenoxylate/atropine (Lomotil)** is available. Bismuth's "**subsalicylate**" is very similar to aspirin (acetyl**salicylic** acid) and should not be used in young children for fear of Reye's syndrome.

Constipation may come from opioid or calcium channel blocker use which blocks calcium from getting to the bowel's smooth muscle. **Polyethylene glycol (Miralax)** can be used, but often a stool softener like **docusate sodium (Colace)** is all a patient needs.

ANTI-NAUSEA (ANTI-EMETICS)
ONDANSETRON (Zofran)
"on-DAN-se-tron" (ZO-fran)
Zofran uses "**z**" o, r, & n from **o**ndanset**r**o**n,** so your nausea will be gone.

PROMETHAZINE (Phenergan)
"pro-METH-ugh-zeen" (FEN-er-gan)
Phenergan will de-**phen**d you until your nausea's **gan**. (gone)

ANTI-DIARRHEALS
BISMUTH SUBSALICYLATE (Pepto-Bismol)
"BIZ-muth sub-Sal-IS-uh-late" (pep-TOE BIZ-mol)
Pepto helps with **pept**ic stuff using **bis**muth.

DIPHENOXYLATE/ATROPINE (Lomotil)
"dye-fen-OX-ill-ate / AT-row-peen" (LOW-moat-ill)
Lomotil slows the bowel's **motil**ity and alleviates diarrhea.

LOPERAMIDE (Imodium)
"Low-PER-uh-mide" (eh-MOE-Dee-um)
Imodium immobilizes the bowel's **mod**e of transport.

CONSTIPATION – OSMOTIC
POLYETHYLENE GLYCOL (Miralax)
"pa-Lee-ETH-ill-een GLY-call" (MIR-uh-lacks)
It's a **miracle** how good you feel after **Miralax**.

CONSTIPATION – STOOL SOFTENER
DOCUSATE SODIUM (Colace)
"DOCK-you-sate SEWED-e-um" (CO-lace)
Docusate improves the **col**on's **pace**, pulls water in, but doesn't race.

III. AUTOIMMUNE DISORDERS

Ulcerative colitis is an autoimmune disease where the body attacks itself. Ulcerative colitis means there is ulceration and inflammation (-itis) in the colon. **Mesalamine (Asacol)** and anti-inflammatory and immunosuppressive drugs are used for this condition.

ULCERATIVE COLITIS
MESALAMINE (Asacol)
"meh-SAL-uh-mean" (AS-uh-call)
Asacol assuages **a col**on with 5-**ASA,** easing a colon's pain today.

Gastrointestinal Drug Quiz (Level 1)

Classify these drugs by placing the corresponding drug class letter next to each medication:

1. Calcium carbonate (Tums)
2. Ranitidine (Zantac)
3. Docusate sodium (Colace)
4. Famotidine (Pepcid)
5. Esomeprazole (Nexium)
6. Loperamide (Imodium)
7. Magnesium hydroxide (Milk of Magnesia)
8. Mesalamine (Asacol)
9. Omeprazole (Prilosec)
10. Ondansetron (Zofran)

Gastrointestinal drug classes:

A. Antacid
B. Anti-diarrheal
C. Anti-nausea
D. Constipation
E. H_2 blocker
F. Proton pump inhibitor
G. Ulcerative colitis

GASTROINTESTINAL DRUG QUIZ (LEVEL 2)

Classify these drugs by placing the corresponding drug class letter next to each medication:

1. Bismuth
2. Diphenoxylate/atropine
3. Pantoprazole
4. Polyethylene glycol
5. Promethazine
6. Calcium carbonate
7. Famotidine
8. Docusate
9. Loperamide
10. Ranitidine

Gastrointestinal drug classes:

A. Antacid
B. Anti-diarrheal
C. Anti-nausea
D. Constipation
E. H_2 blocker
F. Proton pump inhibitor
G. Ulcerative colitis

CHAPTER 2 MUSCULOSKELETAL

I. NSAIDs AND PAIN

Non-steroidal anti-inflammatory drugs (NSAIDs) are named that way because many times steroids are used to treat inflammatory conditions and these medications are different. A few NSAIDs such as **aspirin (Ecotrin)** and **ibuprofen (Motrin)** [taken up to 4 times daily] and **naproxen (Aleve)** [taken twice daily] are available over-the-counter and are meant for intermittent pain or conditions that do not require a medical doctor's attention. **Meloxicam (Mobic)** [once daily] is not OTC. A drug that relieves pain is called an **analgesic**; one that reduces fever is called an **antipyretic**.

The prescription NSAIDs can be used for specific reasons as prescribed by a doctor such as closing an arterial hole (*patent ductus arteriosus*) in a preemie, longer-term relief of pain and inflammation, and so forth. You may hear about cyclooxygenase (COX), an enzyme, and what's important is that a COX-2 inhibitor, like **celecoxib (Celebrex)** is supposed to protect against ulcers.

The question that often comes to the pharmacy is when to use **acetaminophen (Tylenol)** and when to use an **NSAID**. If the patient has inflammation, the acetaminophen will not help. However, if the patient has pain or fever, then either would be appropriate.

ANALGESICS – NSAIDs – COX-1 INHIBITORS

ASPIRIN [ASA] (Ecotrin)
"AS-per-in" (ECK-oh-trin)
Ecotrin is **e**nteric **co**ated aspi**rin**, helps a patient's blood stay thin.

IBUPROFEN (Motrin)
"eye-byou-PRO-fin" (MO-trin)
Motrin works like aspi**rin**, cools a headache, drops a fever's vim.

NAPROXEN (Aleve)
"nap-ROCKS-in" (uh-LEAVE)
Aleve alleviates pain from strains and sprains.

MELOXICAM (Mobic)
"mel-OX-eh-kam" (MO-bik)
Mobic reduces what's inflamed and you only take it once a day!

ANALGESICS – NSAIDS – COX-2 INHIBITORS
CELECOXIB (Celebrex)
"sell-eh-COCKS-ib" (SELL-eh-breks)
Celebrex lets you **celebrate** relief from inflammatory grief.

ANALGESIC – NON-NARCOTIC
ACETAMINOPHEN [APAP] (Tylenol)
"uh-seat-uh-MIN-no-fin" (TIE-Len-all)
Tylenol is the chemical N-acetyl-para-amino-phenol, that's a mouthful to say it all.

II. OPIOIDS AND NARCOTICS

Opioids are very effective pain relievers (**analgesics**), but they do have the potential for addiction. In the past, some small amounts of **codeine** products were available from the pharmacist directly for patients with a serious cough, but this practice has, for the most part, been discontinued.

The physician will determine which analgesic is best for the particular condition and for how long. Often you will hear about drug schedules and these medications. The **drug schedule** is the DEA's (Drug Enforcement Agency) way of categorizing the addictive potential of the drugs.

Drugs that are *schedule I* are illegal and of no medical value such as **heroin**. *Schedule II* drugs are potentially addicting such as **fentanyl (Duragesic), morphine, oxycodone (OxyIR)** by itself, and **oxycodone/APAP (Percocet)**. *Schedule III* drugs are less addicting and include **hydrocodone/APAP (Vicodin)** and **acetaminophen (APAP)/codeine (Tylenol with codeine)**. *Schedule IV* drugs include some sleeping pills such as **zolpidem (Ambien)** and *schedule V* are often cough medicines that include **codeine**, but this is not codeine alone.

OPIOID ANALGESICS – SCHEDULE II

FENTANYL (Duragesic)
"FEN-ta-nil" (dur-uh-GEE-zic)
Duragesic is a long **dura**tion anal**gesic**, sometimes in a patch or on a stick.

MORPHINE
"MORE-feen"
Morphine named after the god of dreams, **Morpheus** to the Greeks or so it seems.

OXYCODONE (OxyIR/Oxycontin)
"ox-e-CO-done" (ox-E-eye-are)
OxyIR is immediate release, for some quick relief.

OXYCODONE/ACETAMINOPHEN (Endocet)
"ox-e-CO-done/ uh-seat-uh-MIN-no-fin" (EN-doe-set)
Endocet is Endo pharmaceuticals' version of **Percocet**, from **acet**aminophen comes the cet.

OPIOID ANALGESICS - SCHEDULE III

HYDROCODONE/ACETAMINOPHIN (Vicodin)
"high-droe-CO-done/uh-seat-uh-MIN-no-fin" (VIE-co-din)
Vicodin combines hydro**cod**one, a codeine derivative, and aceta-minoph**en** you know.

ACETAMINOPHEN WITH CODEINE (Tylenol with Codeine)
"uh-seat-uh-MIN-no-fin with CO-dean"(TIE-Len-all with CO-dean)
Tylenol and **codeine** makes a pair, to reduce cough or pain, to make you feel fair.

NON-OPIOID ANALGESICS - UNSCHEDULED

*****TRAMADOL** (Ultram)
"TRAM-uh-doll" (ULL-tram)
Ultram is **ultra**-pain-relieving **tram**adol, how the generic's called.
Tramadol (Ultram) weakly affects opioid receptors.

III. HEADACHES AND MIGRAINES

Common drugs for headache and migraine include the NSAIDs, **acetaminophen (Tylenol)**, opioids, and the triptans. NSAIDs such as **aspirin (Ecotrin) (ASA)** make sense because they reduce inflammation and one cause of headache is thought to be a swelling of the vessels in the brain. **Acetaminophen (Tylenol)** is a pain reliever and also makes sense. **Caffeine** seems like a strange drug to have in a headache preparation, but caffeine is a potent vasoconstrictor (makes blood vessels narrower) and it is thought to narrow swollen vessels in the brain.

Triptan, the suffix of the drugs in a **5-HT receptor agonist** class such as **sumatriptan (Imitrex)**, work by activating receptors that reduce swelling associated with migraines. They are called *triptans* because two syllables, the last in the generic names of these drugs, are easier to say than **5-hydroxytryptamine receptor agonists.**

MIGRAINE – OTC – NSAID/NON-NARCOTIC ANALGESIC
ASPIRIN/ACETAMINOPHEN/CAFFEINE (Excedrin Migraine)
"AS-per-in/uh-seat-uh-MINnow-fin/ka-FEEN" (ECKS-said-rin)
Excedrin migraine's three ingredients will **exce**ptionally ease the pain that plagues your **brain**.

MIGRAINE – RX - 5-HT RECEPTOR AGONIST (-TRIPTAN)
SUMATRIPTAN (Imitrex)
"Sue-ma-TRIP-tan" (IM-eh-treks)
Sumatriptan trips another migraine run, so you can feel better all at once.

IV. DMARDS AND RHEUMATOID ARTHRITIS

DMARDs stands for **d**isease-**m**odifying **a**ntirheumatic **d**rugs, which means they work against **rheumatoid arthritis**, an autoimmune disorder. These drugs reduce the progression of the disease as opposed to the treatment of **osteoarthritis**, a condition where the body has worn down and the joints are inflamed. Both conditions respond to anti-inflammatories through the use of NSAIDs (non-steroidal anti-inflammatory drugs) such as **ibuprofen (Motrin)** or **aspirin (ASA)**. Glucocorticoids, such as **prednisone (Deltasone),**

can further help reduce inflammation. Special immune-suppressing drugs called DMARDs like **etanercept (Enbrel)** and **methotrexate (Rheumatrex)** are used for autoimmune diseases.

DMARDs

ETANERCEPT (Enbrel)
"eh-TAN-er-sept" (EN-brell)
Etanercept enables arthritic **rel**ief, from an autoimmune disease.

METHOTREXATE (Rheumatrex)
"meth-oh-TREKS-ate"(ROOM-uh-treks)
Meth o T-Rex ate the rheumatic inflammate.

V. OSTEOPOROSIS

Do not to confuse *osteoarthritis*, a joint disease, with *osteoporosis*, which is a thinning in the density of the bone tissue. Drugs for **osteoporosis** build the bone back up. Because bone growth is slow, certain drugs like **alendronate (Fosamax)** can be given weekly or **ibandronate (Boniva)** can be given monthly.

OSTEOPOROSIS – BISPHOSPHONATE (-DRONATE)

ALENDRONATE (Fosamax)
"uh-LEN-dro-Nate" (FA-seh-max)
Fosamax replaces **bone fossa** to the **max,** wait 30 minutes before you lie down to relax.

IBANDRONATE (Boniva)
"eh-BAND-row-Nate" (bo-KNEE-vuh)
Boniva returns **bone's** life or **vida** if Spanish is your spice.

VI. GOUT

Gout is considered an acute inflammatory arthritis that can be treated acutely (right away) with an NSAID such as **ibuprofen (Motrin)** or **colchicine (Cholcrys)**. Colchicine is very hard on the stomach and can only be used for a few doses.

Gout can also be treated prophylactically (doing something to prevent the recurrence) with a drug that helps reduce uric acid, a major component in the crystals that cause the gouty pain. Drugs that alter uric acid levels include **allopurinol (Zyloprim)** and **febuxostat (Uloric).**

ANTI-GOUT – *FOR ACUTE ATTACKS*
COLCHICINE (Cholcrys)
"COAL-che-seen" (COAL-Chris)
Cholcrys helps clear gouty **crystals,** in big toes and other places.

ANTI-GOUT – *URIC ACID REDUCERS*
ALLOPURINOL (Zyloprim)
"aloe-PURE-in-all" (ZY-low-prim)
Zyloprim lowers uric acid to **pre**vent a gouty torrent.

FEBUXOSTAT (Uloric)
"fe-BUCKS-oh-stat" (YOU-lore-ick)
Uloric helps yo**u lo**wer **uric** acid levels, helping fight the gout devil.

MUSCULOSKELETAL DRUG QUIZ (LEVEL 1)

Classify these drugs by placing the corresponding drug class letter next to each medication:

1. Acetaminophen (Tylenol)
2. Alendronate (Fosamax)
3. ASA/APAP/caffeine (Excedrin)
4. Colchicine (Colcrys)
5. Etanercept (Enbrel)
6. Fentanyl (Duragesic)
7. Hydrocodone/APAP (Vicodin)
8. Ibuprofen (Motrin)
9. Celecoxib (Celebrex)
10. Sumatriptan (Imitrex)

Musculoskeletal Drug Classes:

A. 5-HT receptor agonist for headache
B. Anti-gout
C. Bisphosphonate for osteoporosis
D. DMARD
E. Non-narcotic analgesic - single
F. Non-narcotic analgesic combo - headache
G. NSAID COX-1
H. NSAID COX-2
I. Opioid analgesic

MUSCULOSKELETAL DRUG QUIZ (LEVEL 2)

Classify these drugs by placing the corresponding drug class letter next to each medication:

1. Methotrexate
2. Morphine
3. Oxycodone
4. Naproxen
5. Febuxostat
6. Ibandronate
7. Allopurinol
8. Aspirin
9. Alendronate
10. APAP/Codeine

Musculoskeletal Drug Classes:

A. 5-HT receptor agonist for headache
B. Anti-gout
C. Bisphosphonate for osteoporosis
D. DMARD
E. Non-narcotic analgesic - single
F. Non-narcotic analgesic combo - headache
G. NSAID COX-1
H. NSAID COX-2
I. Opioid analgesic

CHAPTER 3 RESPIRATORY

I. ANTIHISTAMINES

Antihistamines are divided into two generations: First and second. The first and older generation would make patients sleepy. Drugs such as **diphenhydramine (Benadryl)** are still used as antihistamines and also as an over-the-counter sleep aid. The new generation cannot pass through the blood-brain barrier and into the central nervous system and cause no or minimal drowsiness. Drugs in this second generation include **cetirizine (Zyrtec)** and **loratadine (Claritin)**.

ANTIHISTAMINE – 1ST GENERATION
DIPHENHYDRAMINE (Benadryl)
"dye-fen-HIGH-dra-mean" (BEN-uh-drill)
Benadryl benefits you by **dry**ing up your runny nose.

ANTIHISTAMINE – 2ND GENERATION
CETIRIZINE (Zyrtec)
"seh-TIRE-uh-zine" (ZEER-tech)
Zyrtec provides **"z" tech**nical allergy relief all year.

LORATADINE (Claritin)
"lore-AT-uh-dean" (KLAR-eh-tin)
Claritin clears allergy symptoms, so go outside and breathe air **in**.

II. COUGH AND ALLERGIC RHINITIS

Cough can be prevented with an over-the-counter medication **guaifenesin with dextromethorphan (Robitussin DM)**. The **guaifenesin** is a mucolytic, or something that breaks up (-lytic) mucous (muco-) and chest congestion and the **dextromethorphan** is the cough suppressant. In severe cases, a **codeine**-based product such as **guaifenesin/codeine (Cheratussin AC)** may be used. Allergic rhinitis is an inflammation (-itis) of the nose (rhin-), and is treated with a local steroid like **mometasone (Nasonex).**

MUCOLYTIC/COUGH SUPPRESSANT – OTC

GUAIFENESIN/DEXTROMETHORPHAN (Robitussin DM)
"gwhy-FEN-uh-sin/decks-trow-meh-THOR-fan" (row-bi-TUSS-in)
Robitussin robs your cough so at bedtime you don't **tuss**le.

MUCOLYTIC/COUGH SUPPRESSANT – RX

GUAIFENESIN/CODEINE (Cheratussin AC)
"gwhy-FEN-uh-sin/CO-dean" (CHAIR-ugh-tuss-in)
Cheratussin AC is good if you're hacking up, you see.

ALLERGIC RHINITIS – NASAL STEROID (-SONE)

MOMETASONE (Nasonex)
"Moe-MET-uh-sewn" (NEIGH-zo-nex)
Nasonex keeps your nose from sneezing and wheezing.

III. ASTHMA

Asthma can be thought of as a disease of inflammation and bronchoconstriction (the lung's branches tighten). Oral steroids such as **methylprednisolone (Medrol)** and **prednisone (Deltasone)** are used to help reduce lung inflammation when a severe attack has happened. For immediate relief during an attack, albuterol (**ProAir HFA, Ventolin HFA**) is the short acting bronchodilator that will reverse the bronchoconstriction.

The products **fluticasone/salmeterol (Advair)** or **budesonide/formoterol (Symbicort)** will provide relief from both inflammation and bronchoconstriction by combining a steroid and long acting bronchodilator. Notice that most steroids end or have – sone in the name and that bronchodilators have –terol in the suffix.

Tiotropium (Spiriva) is considered an anticholinergic medication. Often these medications cause dry mouth, constipation and other unwanted adverse effects. However, **tiotropium (Spiriva)** affects the smooth muscle of the lungs, allowing for bronchodilation and relaxation. Expect the suffix –tropium with these medications.

Montelukast (Singulair) inhibits leukotriene receptors. Leukotrienes are important in the process of bronchoconstriction, which is usually a process that helps protect the lungs against foreign contaminants. Drugs in this class end in –lukast.

ASTHMA – ORAL STEROIDS (-SONE/-LONE)

METHYLPREDNISOLONE (Medrol)
"meth-ill-pred-NISS-uh-lone" (MED-rol)
Medrol can come in a pack of six days and twenty-one pills, and then you'll be off your back.

PREDNISONE (Deltasone)
"PRED-ni-sewn" (DEALT-uh-sewn)
Prednisone eases asthma inflammation for good respiration.

ASTHMA – SHORT-ACTING BETA AGONIST (-TEROL)

ALBUTEROL (ProAir)
"Al-BYOU-ter-all" (PRO-air)
ProAir provides **air** to asthmatics, so they can do gymnastics.

ASTHMA – STEROID/LONG-ACTING BRONCHODILATOR

BUDESONIDE/FORMOTEROL (Symbicort)
"byou-DES-uh-nide/four-MOE-ter-all" (SIM-buh-court)
Symicort is **symbiotic**, two drugs for asthma, and you might try it.

FLUTICASONE/SALMETEROL (Advair)
"flue-TIC-uh-sewn/Sal-MEET-er-all" (ADD-vair)
Advair adds two drugs to reduce an asthmatic's **air**flow plugs.

ASTHMA/COPD – ANTI-CHOLINERGIC (-TROPIUM)

TIOTROPIUM (Spiriva)
"tie-oh-TROW-pee-um"(Spur-EE-va)
Spiriva lasts all day, lets you breathe, go out and play.

ASTHMA – LEUKOTRIENE RECEPTOR ANTAGONIST (-LUKAST)

MONTELUKAST (Singulair)
"Monte-LUKE-ast" (SING-you-lair)
Singulair a **single** time a day, to improve **air**flow, so kids can play.

IV. Nasal Congestion and Anaphylaxis

Nasal decongestants like **pseudoephedrine (Sudafed)** constrict blood vessels in the nose and sinuses, reducing the amount of mucus. Anaphylaxis is a special type of over-reaction of the body to something like an insect bite or bee sting. **Epinephrine (EpiPen)** quickly reverses the effects, keeping the airway open.

Congestion – Decongestant

PSEUDOEPHEDRINE (Sudafed)
"Sue-doe-uh-FED-ran" (Sue-duh-FED)
Sudafed is short for **pseudoephed**rine, which will clear up your congestion.

Anaphylaxis

EPINEPHRINE (EpiPen)
"eh-pee-NEF-rin" (EP-e-pen)
EpiPen can save an anaphylactic patient from a **pen**icillin allergy with an **epi**nephrine **pen** in a hurry.

RESPIRATORY DRUG QUIZ (LEVEL 1)

Classify these drugs by placing the corresponding drug class letter next to each medication:

1. Albuterol (ProAir)
2. Cetirizine (Zyrtec)
3. Diphenhydramine (Benadryl)
4. Fluticasone/salmeterol (Advair)
5. Guaifenesin/DM (Robitussin DM)
6. Tiotropium (Spiriva)
7. Loratadine (Claritin)
8. Montelukast (Singulair)
9. Pseudoephedrine (Sudafed)
10. Methylprednisolone (Medrol)

Respiratory drug classes:

A. 1st-generation antihistamine
B. 2nd-generation antihistamine
C. Anticholinergic
D. Decongestant
E. Leukotriene receptor antagonist
F. Mucolytic/cough suppressant
G. Oral steroid
H. Nasal steroid
I. Short-acting bronchodilator
J. Steroid/long-acting bronchodilator

Respiratory Drug Quiz (Level 2)

Classify these drugs by placing the corresponding drug class letter next to each medication:

1. Budesonide/formoterol
2. Guaifenesin/codeine
3. Mometasone
4. Fluticasone/salmeterol
5. Pseudoephedrine
6. Cetirizine
7. Diphenhydramine
8. Albuterol
9. Montelukast
10. Prednisone

Respiratory drug classes:

A. 1st-generation antihistamine
B. 2nd-generation antihistamine
C. Anticholinergic
D. Decongestant
E. Leukotriene receptor antagonist
F. Mucolytic/cough suppressant
G. Oral steroid
H. Nasal steroid
I. Short-acting bronchodilator
J. Steroid/long-acting bronchodilator

CHAPTER 4 IMMUNE

I. ANTIMICROBIALS IN A NUTSHELL

Antimicrobials can be divided into **antibiotics** (drugs for bacteria), **antifungals** (drugs for mycoses or fungi), or **antivirals**, (drugs for viruses). I'm not going to review all the different ways these drugs can work, I just want to show how, in this particular class of drugs, prefixes and suffixes are especially prevalent.

Suffixes:
>   **-azole** – Antifungal [do not confuse with -prazole]
>   **-cillin** – Penicillin antibiotic
>   **-cycline** – Tetracycline antibiotic
>   **-floxacin** – Fluoroquinolone antibiotic
>   **-micin, mycin** – Possible aminoglycoside antibiotic
>   [not *-thromycin*]
>   **-thromycin** – Macrolide antibiotic
>   **-vir** – Antiviral

Prefixes:
>   **Sulfa-** Sulfa antibiotic.
>   **Cef-, Ceph-** Cephalosporin antibiotic

II. PENICILLINS, CEPHALOSPORINS, MACROLIDES

Penicillins were one of the first antimicrobial classes to appear. Sometimes we see resistance to a single antibiotic like **amoxicillin (Amoxil)**. **Amoxicillin/clavulanate (Augmentin)** adds clavulanate to protect the amoxicillin against an enzyme bacteria produce called a beta-lactamase. It is named after the chemical structure (a beta lactam) that is in all penicillins

Cephalosporins can have cross-sensitivity with penicillins. Patients who are allergic to one may be allergic to the other. Cephalosporins are classified into generations. The first-generation drugs such as **cephalexin (Keflex)** do not penetrate the cerebrospinal fluid (CSF), have poor gram-negative bacterial coverage (a gram-negative bacteria will not take up a gram stain and has an extra protective layer), and are subject to beta-lactamases. As we move to third-generation **ceftriaxone (Rocephin)** and fourth-generation **cefepime (Maxipime)** we get good penetration into the CSF, have good gram-negative coverage and resistance to beta lactamases.

Macrolides, are sometimes called "erythromycins" after the original drug in the class. **Erythromycin (E-Mycin)** may have to be taken up to four times a day, **clarithromycin (Biaxin)** twice a day (notice the bi- prefix) and **azithromycin (Zithromax)** only has to be taken once a day, though most schedules include a double dose of azithromycin on the first day and a single dose the following four days. The double dose is called a loading dose.

ANTIBIOTICS: PENICILLINS
AMOXICILLIN (Amoxil)
"uh-mocks-eh-SILL-in" (uh-MOCKS-ill)
Amoxil is from **amoxi**cillin, to bacteria's wall it does the ki**llin**'.

ANTIBIOTICS: PENICILLIN/BETA-LACTAMASE INHIBITOR
AMOXICILLIN/CLAVULANATE (Augmentin)
"uh-mocks-eh-SILL-in/clav-you-LAWN-ate" (og-MENT-in)
Augmentin augments amoxicill**in**'s defense against a beta-lactamase offense.

ANTIBIOTICS: CEPHALOSPORINS (CEF-/CEPH-)
CEPHALEXIN (Keflex)
"sef-uh-LEX-in" (KE-flecks)
Keflex is a first-generation bacterial **k**iller, uses letters from **cephalex**in to make its name.

CEFTRIAXONE (Rocephin)
"sef-try-AX-own" (row-SEF-in)
Rocephin is Hoffman-La**Ro**che's patent, a third-generation **ceph**alosporin antibacterial combatant.

CEFEPIME (Maxipime)
"SEF-eh-peem" (MAX-eh-peem)
Maxipime is the fourth and **max** generation, of generic cefe**pime**.

ANTIBIOTICS: MACROLIDES (-THROMYCIN)

ERYTHROMYCIN (E-Mycin)
"err-ITH-row-my-sin" (E-MY-sin)
E-mycin is short for the generic erythro**mycin** that puts up a fight against bacterial invasion.

CLARITHROMYCIN (Biaxin)
"Claire-ITH-row-my-sin" (bi-AX-in)
Biaxin is like erythromycin, but given **b.i.d.**, or half as often.

AZITHROMYCIN (Zithromax)
"a-ZITH-row-my-sin" (ZITH-row-max)
Zithromax uses the generic a**zithro**mycin's letters, to provide **max**imum antibiotic coverage.

III. ANTIBIOTICS: FLUOROQUINOLONES, TETRACYCLINES

AMINOGLYCOSIDES

Fluoroquinolones are sometimes named "floxacins" after their suffix. **Tetracyclines** are named after the four (tetra-) member chemical ring (-cycline). Both have some similarities in their adverse effect profiles. For example, both classes of drugs cause photosensitivity (an increased sensitivity to burning from sunlight) and chelation (a binding with cations such as the Ca^{++} in milk or antacids). Fluoroquinolones also have a very unique side effect in that sometimes they can cause tendon rupture, although rarely. **Aminoglycosides** are notorious for damaging the kidneys (nephrotoxicity) and ears (ototoxicity).

ANTIBIOTICS: FLUOROQUINOLONES (-FLOXACIN)

CIPROFLOXACIN (Cipro)
"sip-row-FLOCKS-uh-sin" (SIP-row)
Cipro's brand name cuts the –floxacin from **cipro**floxacin.

LEVOFLOXACIN (Levaquin)
"Lee-vo-FLOCKS-uh-sin" (LEV-uh-Quinn)
Levaquin is the brand name for the fluoro**quin**olone antibiotic **levo**floxacin.

ANTIBIOTICS: TETRACYCLINES (-CYCLINE)

DOXYCYCLINE (Doryx)
"docks-e-SIGH-clean" (DOOR-icks)
Doryx is **doxy**cycline, sure is a tetracycline.

TETRACYCLINE (Sumycin)
"tet-rah-SIGH-clean" (Sue-MY-sin)
Tetracycline has four rings, to give bacteria a big sting.

ANTIBIOTICS: AMINOGLYCOSIDES

AMIKACIN (Amikin)
"am-eh-KAY-sin" (AM-eh-kin)
Amikin takes a prefix and suffix from **amik**acin, an aminoglycoside bacteria don't want to find themselves facin'.

GENTAMICIN (Garamycin)
"Jenn-ta-MY-sin" (gare-uh-MY-sin)
Garamycin is short for **gentamicin** spelled with **my** not **-icin**.

IV. ANTIBIOTICS: OTHER CLASSES

Some antibiotics do not fit neatly into a classification, or there is only one drug in the class.

Clindamycin (Cleocin) is often used for dental prophylaxis when a patient is penicillin allergic or for severe acne. When used orally it can cause a severe condition known as pseudomembranous colitis, also known as antibiotic associated diarrhea (AAD).

Metronidazole (Flagyl) is used for various infections including *H. Pylori* as part of triple therapy. A notable side effect of metronidazole is the disulfiram reaction where a patient may projectile vomit if metronidazole is combined with alcohol.

Sulfamethoxazole/trimethoprim (Bactrim) is a combination therapy that affects the folic acid in bacteria. Humans can ingest folic acid so it does not affect us adversely. However, sulfa medications can sometimes cause allergic reactions. Sulfa drugs are usually used for urinary tract infections (UTIs) and prophylaxis (prevention) of certain infections associated with immunocompromised patients such as HIV patients. Sulfamethoxazole can cause a rare, but life threatening condition known as Stevens-Johnson syndrome.

Vancomycin (Vancocin) is sometimes the last line of defense against deadly bacterial infections and often there is a special protocol as to who can and cannot get vancomycin. Vancomycin can cause a hypersensitivity reaction called red man syndrome.

ANTIBIOTICS: LINCOSAMIDE
CLINDAMYCIN (Cleocin)
"clin-duh-MY-sin" (KLEE-oh-sin)
Cleocin is short for **clindamycin**, clears up acne so you can grin.

ANTIBIOTICS: NITROIMIDAZOLE / ANTI-PROTOZOAL
METRONIDAZOLE (Flagyl)
"met-ruh-NID-uh-zole" (FLADGE-ill)
Flagyl is the nitroimidazole pill, with almost all the letters of metronidazole, that kills *Clostridium **difficile**.*

ANTIBIOTICS: DIHIDROFOLATE REDUCTASE INHIBITOR (SULFA-)
SULFAMETHOXAZOLE/TRIMETHOPRIM (SMZ-TMP) "sull-fa-meth-OX-uh-zole/try-METH-oh-prim" (s-m-zee/tee-m-pee)
SMZ/TMP is the acronym for the sulfamethoxazole/trimethoprim, a mouthful to say, but it will clear your urine and save the day.

ANTIBIOTICS: GLYCOPEPTIDE
VANCOMYCIN (Vancocin)
"van-co-MY-sin" (VAN-co-sin)
Vancocin will **vanquish** MRSA, a last resort; we don't always give it away.

V. TUBERCULOSIS
Antituberculosis agents are generally used for an extended period of time (months) and more than one drug is used to prevent resistance because tuberculosis is a very slow growing microbe.

ETHAMBUTOL (Myambutol)
"eh-THAM-byou-tall" (my-AM-byou-tall)
Myambutol is the **my**cobacterium fighting TB drug eth**ambutol**.

ISONIAZID (INH)
"eye-sew-NIGH-uh-zid" (EYE-en-h)
INH is an acronym for **i**s**o**nicoti**n**yl**h**ydrazine, a TB drug's name,
few longer we've seen.

PYRAZINAMIDE (PZA)
"pier-uh-ZIN-uh-mide" (pee-zee-a)
PZA is the acronym for the TB drug **p**yra**z**in**a**mide.

RIFAMPIN (Rifadin)
"rif-AMP-in" (rif-UH-din)
Rifandin is short for generic **rif**amp**in**, will turn your pee orange.

VI. FUNGI

Antifungals are divided into two types, those that are systemic (in the
body) and those that are dermatologic (on the skin). Before the
advent of antifungals, most systemic fungal infections were deadly.

Amphotericin B (Fungizone) is often used for systemic infections
and **nystatin (Mycostatin)** is used for thrush or yeast infections.

AMPHOTERICIN B (Fungizone)
"am-foe-TER-uh-sin Bee" (FUN-gah-zone)
Fungizone kills systemic **fungi**, but watch your kidney **zone**.

FLUCONAZOLE (Diflucan)
"flue-CON-uh-zole" (die-FLUE-can)
Diflucan uses the first two syllables of **flucon**azole, to kill fungi,
that's its role.

NYSTATIN (Mycostatin)
"NIGH-stat-in" (MY-co-stat-in)
Mycostatin uses the suffix from **nystatin**, the generic name and prefix **myco**, meaning fungus.

VII. VIRUSES

Antivirals are often named after the virus they are trying to kill. Many antivirals have "vir" in the middle or end of the generic and/or brand name.

ANTIVIRALS – INFLUENZA (-VIR)

Drugs for the flu such as **oseltamivir (Tamiflu)** and **zanamivir (Relenza)** both need to be taken within 48 hours of the infection to work properly.

OSELTAMIVIR (Tamiflu)
"owe-sell-TAM-eh-veer" (TA-mi-flue)
Tamiflu tames in**flu**enza.

ZANAMIVIR (Relenza)
"za-NAH-mi-veer" (rah-LEN-zuh)
Relenza represses in**flu**enza virus and that is desirous.

ANTIVIRALS – HERPES (-VIR)

Drugs for herpes infections such as **acyclovir (Zovirax)** and **valacyclovir (Valtrex)** can help prevent recurrences and treat an infection, but they will not cure the disease.

ACYCLOVIR (Zovirax)
"a-SIGH-clo-veer" (zo-VIE-racks)
Zovirax axes **z**oster **vir**us.

VALACYCLOVIR (Valtrex)
"Val-uh-SIGH-clo-veer" (VAL-trex)
Valtrex is **val**acyclovir plus **t-rex,** and wrecks a virus.

ANTIVIRALS – HIV (-VIR)

A drug for HIV such as **zidovudine (Retrovir)** affects specific targets in the cell or retrovirus. HIV medications, like tuberculosis medications, are used in combination.

ZIDOVUDINE (Retrovir)
"zie-DOE-view-dean" (REH-tro-veer)
Retrovir kills **retrovir**uses like HIV, with these drugs, you need 3.

Classify these drugs by placing the corresponding drug class letter next to each medication:

1. Amoxicillin (Amoxil)
2. Azithromycin (Zithromax)
3. Cefepime (Maxipime)
4. Ceftriaxone (Rocephin)
5. Fluconazole (Diflucan)
6. Gentamicin (Garamycin)
7. Isoniazid (INH)
8. Levofloxacin (Levaquin)
9. Nystatin (Mycostatin)
10. Valacyclovir (Valtrex)

Immune drug classes:

A. 1st generation cephalosporin
B. 2nd generation cephalosporin
C. 3rd generation cephalosporin
D. 4th generation cephalosporin
E. Antibiotic: aminoglycoside
F. Antibiotic: fluoroquinolone
G. Antibiotic: macrolide
H. Antibiotic: penicillin
I. Antibiotic: sulfa
J. Antibiotic: tetracycline
K. Anti-fungal
L. Anti-tuberculosis
M. Anti-viral (herpes)
N. Anti-viral (HIV)
O. Anti-viral (influenza)

IMMUNE DRUG QUIZ (LEVEL 2)

Classify these drugs by placing the corresponding drug class letter next to each medication:

1. Rifampin
2. Amphotericin B
3. Amikacin
4. Ciprofloxacin
5. Pyrazinamide
6. Acyclovir
7. Cephalexin
8. SMZ/TMP
9. Erythromycin
10. Oseltamivir

Immune drug classes:

A. 1st generation cephalosporin
B. 2nd generation cephalosporin
C. 3rd generation cephalosporin
D. 4th generation cephalosporin
E. Antibiotic: aminoglycoside
F. Antibiotic: fluoroquinolone
G. Antibiotic: macrolide
H. Antibiotic: penicillin
I. Antibiotic: sulfa
J. Antibiotic: tetracycline
K. Anti-fungal
L. Anti-tuberculosis
M. Anti-viral (herpes)
N. Anti-viral (HIV)
O. Anti-viral (influenza)

CHAPTER 5 NEURO

I. SEDATIVE-HYPNOTICS (SLEEPING PILLS)

Sedative-hypnotics help patients sleep. Although benzodiazepines such as **clonazepam (Klonopin), diazepam (Valium)**, and **lorazepam (Ativan)** as well as the over-the-counter antihistamine **diphenhydramine (Benadryl)** can also be used to help patients sleep, those medications are discussed in other sections. Most sedative-hypnotics have a hint towards their function in their brand names: **Eszopiclone (Lunesta)** with Luna for "moon", **ramelton (Rozerem)** refers to REM sleep, and **zolpidem (Ambien)** creates an ambient (tranquil) environment.

SEDATIVE-HYPNOTICS

ESZOPICLONE (Lunesta)
"es-zo-PEH-clone" (Lou-NES-tuh)
Lunesta uses the Latin for moon (**Luna**) so you can **rest – ahhhh.**

RAMELTON (Rozerem)
"ram-ELL-tawn" (row-ZER-em)
Rozerem helps you get **REM** (rapid eye movement) sleep and your **z**'s, with that, you must be pleased.

TRAZODONE (Desyrel)
"TRAYS-uh-dohn" (DEZ-er-ill)
Desyrel will help you sleep and **doze.**

ZOLPIDEM (Ambien)
"ZOLE-pi-dem" (AM-bee-en)
Ambien creates an **ambient**, sleepy environment.

II. FOUR CLASSES OF ANTIDEPRESSANT

Many students are intimidated by the length of the names of the antidepressant drug classes. Break down the word to figure out its function. The **selective serotonin reuptake inhibitors (SSRIs)** include drugs such as **citalopram (Celexa), escitalopram (Lexapro), paroxetine (Paxil), fluoxetine (Prozac)**, and **sertraline**

(Zoloft). This drug will inhibit, or block the reuptake of serotonin. If there is more serotonin around, then the mood should be elevated. Note the escitalopram and citalopram have the same es- prefix discussed in the proton pump inhibitor section.

A similar type of drug is the **serotonin-norepinephrine reuptake inhibitor (SNRI) venlafaxine (Effexor)** that affects two, not one neurotransmitter.

The third group of drugs is named not after the transmitter it affects, but what the chemical structure looks like. A **tricyclic antidepressant (TCA)** has three rings and an example is **amitriptyline (Elavil)**, meant to elevate one's mood.

The last group includes the **monoamine oxidase inhibitors (MAOIs)**. A word that ends in –ase is usually an enzyme, so if an antidepressant blocks the enzyme, then that monoamine neurotransmitter must be a neurotransmitter, elevating mood. An example of an MAOI is **phenelzine (Nardil)**.

SELECTIVE SEROTONIN REUPTAKE INHIBITORS (SSRIs)
CITALOPRAM (Celexa)
"sit-AL-oh-pram" (SELL-ex-uh)
Celexa starts with a "**c**", like the generic citalopram, and can **relax** depression and anxiety.

ESCITALOPRAM (Lexapro)
"es-sit-AL-oh-pram" (LECKS-uh-pro)
Lexapro helps you relax and find solace from despair, that you might feel better in a few weeks there.

FLUOXETINE (Prozac)
"flue-OX-uh-teen" (PRO-Zack)
Prozac provides **exactly** what a depressed patient needs.

PAROXETINE (Paxil)
"par-OX-eh-teen" (PACKS-ill)
Paxil takes **p-a-x-i** from **pa**roxetine.

SERTRALINE (Zoloft)
"SIR-tra-lean" (ZO-loft)
Zoloft lofts a depressed patient's mood.

SEROTONIN-NOREPINEPHRINE REUPTAKE INHIBITORS (SNRIs)

VENLAFAXINE (Effexor)
"VEN-luh-facts-een" (Eff-ECKS-or)
Effexor effects two neurotransmitters, not just serotonin, but norepinephrine as well.

TRICYCLIC ANTIDEPRESSANTS (TCAs)

AMITRIPTYLINE (Elavil)
"ah-meh-TRIP-ta-lean" (Elle-uh-vill)
Elavil can **elevate** your mood.

MONOAMINE OXIDASE INHIBITORS (MAOIs)

ISOCARBOXAZID (Marplan)
"iso-car-BOX-uh-zid" (MAR-plan)
Marplan for the atypical sad man who laments, "I so carve boxes."

PHENELZINE (Nardil)
"FEN-uhl-zine" (NAR-dill)
Nardil's A is in the middle of **M** And **O**, **I** say.

TRANYLCYPROMINE (Parnate)
"tran-ill-SIP-row-mean" (PAR-Nate)
Parnate's great for a mood that needs to elevate.

III. BENZODIAZEPINES

Benzodiazepines are used for anxiety or muscle relaxation. They are named like the tricyclic antidepressants, after their chemical structure which is a combination of a benzene ring and a diazepine ring. Because the word **benzodiazepine** has so many syllables, most people just call them **benzos**. Examples include **alprazolam (Xanax), clonazepam (Klonopin), diazepam (Valium)**, and

lorazepam (Ativan). Note benzodiazepines have similar generic suffixes –zolam and –zepam.

BENZODIAZEPINES (-ZOLAM/–ZEPAM)

ALPRAZOLAM (Xanax)
"Al-PRAY-zo-lam" (ZAN-ax)
Alprazolam has one z, benzodiazepine has two, **Xanax** sounds like a "z", to help you get a snooze and "**x's**" out **anx**iety, too.

CLONAZEPAM (Klonopin)
"klah-NAZ-uh-Pam" (KLON-uh-pin)
Klonopin uses the phonetic spelling of **clonazepam's** prefix -**clon**.

DIAZEPAM (Valium)
"dye-A's-eh-Pam" (VAL-e-um)
Valium helps relax you like the **val**erian root would too.

LORAZEPAM (Ativan)
"lore-A's-eh-Pam" (AT-eh-van)
Ativan is a benzo variety that likes **vanquishing** anxiety.

IV. ADHD MEDICATIONS

ADHD (attention-deficit-hyperactivity disorder) medications, which are stimulants, calm a patient who has a hyperactive mind and/or body without the sedative effect. Examples include **dexme-thylphenidate (Focalin)** and **methylphenidate (Concerta)**.

These two medications have the same root, methylphenidate. In chemistry, compounds also direct plane-polarized light either to the left or right. These terms are either "d" or "(+)" for dextrorotatory compounds rotating plane-polarized light to the right or "l" or "(-)" designating levorotatory compounds rotating plane-polarized light to the left. Thus, the dexmethylphenidate would be expected to rotate plane-polarized light to the right. Dexmethylphenidate is supposed to be either more effective, last longer or have fewer side effects that methylphenidate.

Atomoxetine (Strattera) is a non-stimulant medication and because there is not a potential for abuse, it does not carry a DEA schedule.

ADHD MEDICATIONS – STIMULANT – SCHEDULE II

DEXMETHYLPHENIDATE (Focalin)
"dex-meth-ill-FEN-eh-date" (FOE-ca-lin)
Focalin helps a patient **focus**.

METHYLPHENIDATE (Concerta)
"meth-ill-FEN-eh-date" (con-CERT-uh)
Concerta can help a patient **concentrate**.

ADHD MEDICATIONS – NON-STIMULANT – NON-SCHEDULED

ATOMOXETINE (Strattera)
"a-to-MOCKS-e-teen" (stra-TER-uh)
Strattera helps **stra**ighten patients' **atte**ntion.

V. BIPOLAR

Mood stabilizers such as lithium are especially sensitive to electro-
lyte imbalances. If you look at the periodic table you see that lithium
(Li) and sodium (Na) are in the same group (the alkali metals) and
each have a +1 charge as an ion.

Because of this similarity, what happens to sodium will happen to
lithium causing a toxic or subtherapeutic state if the lithium is
retained or excreted, respectively. Other meds might be needed until
the lithium level is correct.

BIPOLAR DISORDER – SIMPLE SALT

LITHIUM
"LITH-e-um"
Lithium is in the same group as Nat**rium** (Na) – sodium – and where
the salt goeth, the lithium goeth too.

VI. SCHIZOPHRENIA

Medications for schizophrenia are grouped into typical (1st generation) or atypical (2nd generation). The typical antipsychotics such as
chlorpromazine (Thorazine) and **Haloperidol (Haldol)** are further
divided into low potency and high potency, respectively.

While these two antipsychotics have the same therapeutic effect, their side effect profiles are different. Low potency drugs cause more sedation, but fewer extrapyramidal symptoms. High potency drugs cause more extrapyramidal symptoms (movement disorders), but less sedation. The typical antipsychotics are used for positive symptoms such as delusions, hallucinations and paranoia.

Atypical antipsychotics such as **olanzapine (Zyprexa)**, **quetiapine (Seroquel)** and **risperidone (Risperdal)** cause fewer extrapyramidal effects, but more metabolic effects like weight gain, diabetes and hyperlipidemia. These drugs can be used for positive symptoms such as delusions as well as negative symptoms such as poor motivation and emotional and social withdrawal.

SCHIZOPHRENIA – TYPICAL ANTIPSYCHOTIC/LOW POTENCY
CHLORPROMAZINE (Thorazine)
"Klor-PRO-mah-zeen" (THOR-uh-zeen)
Thorazine sometimes causes a shuffle, watch for dry anticholinergic effects, but less EPS.

SCHIZOPHRENIA – TYPICAL ANTIPSYCHOTIC/HIGH POTENCY
HALOPERIDOL (Haldol)
"hal-low-PEAR-eh-doll" (HAL-doll)
Haldol is **hal**operi**dol**, may cause EPS, but less anticholinergic mess.

SCHIZOPHRENIA – ATYPICAL ANTIPSYCHOTIC
OLANZAPINE (Zyprexa)
"oh-LANZ-uh-peen" (ZYE-preks-uh)
Zyprexa is atypical, ya know, less EPS, but metabolic syndrome, oh no.

QUETIAPINE (Seroquel)
"Kweh-TIE-uh-peen" (SEAR-uh-kwell)
Seroquel quells disturbing thoughts, with less EPS, it's worth a shot.

RISPERIDONE (Risperdal)
"ris-PEAR-eh-doen" (RIS-per-doll)
Risperdal is **risper**idone, an antipsychotic that is known.

VII. ANTIEPILEPTICS

The traditional anti-epileptic drugs **carbamazepine (Tegretol)**, **divalproex (Depakote)** and **phenytoin (Dilantin)** have been around for a long time and often we know what to expect with their use.

We may have less experience with the newer anti-epileptics such as **gabapentin (Neurontin)** and **pregabalin (Lyrica)**, but they are just as effective as the traditional drugs. Both groups are tried until a drug is found that matches the seizure profile.

ANTIEPILEPTICS – TRADITIONAL

CARBAMAZEPINE (Tegretol)
"car-bah-MAZE-uh-peen" (TEG-reh-tawl)
Tegretol controls seizures.

DIVALPROEX (Depakote)
"dye-Val-PRO-ex" (DEP-uh-coat)
Depakote controls convulsions, uses five letters from **divalproex**.

PHENYTOIN (Dilantin)
"FEN-eh-toyn" (DYE-lan-tin)
Dilantin uses three letters of phe**n**y**t**o**in**, to stop a patient from shakin'.

ANTIEPILEPTICS – NEWER

GABAPENTIN (Neurontin)
"gab-uh-PEN-tin" (NER-on-tin)
Neurontin affects **neur**onal pulsing, uses the last four letters of gabape**ntin.**

PREGABALIN (Lyrica)
"pre-GAB-uh-lin" (LEER-eh-ca)
Lyrica can put neurons back in **lyric** rhythm and control.

VII. MISCELLANEOUS NEURO MEDICATIONS

Drugs for Alzheimer's, Parkinson's, vertigo, and muscle relaxation are included in this section.

DRUGS FOR ALZHEIMER'S

DONEPEZIL (Aricept)
"Doe-NEP-eh-zill" (ERR-eh-sept)
Aricept improves per**cept**ion and **A**lzheimer's patients' recollection.

MEMANTINE (Namenda)
"Meh-MAN-teen" (Nuh-MEN-duh)
Namenda comes from **NMDA**, the receptor antagonist that will help you remember today.

DRUGS FOR PARKINSON'S

LEVODOPA/CARBIDOPA (Sinemet)
"LEE-vo-doe-pa CAR-bid-oh-pa" (SIN-uh-met)
Sinemet works **syn**ergistically to help Parkinson's patients' tremors cease.

SELEGILINE (Eldepryl)
"se-LEDGE-eh-lean" (EL-duh-pril)
Eldepryl helps with Parkinson's disease, a condition more prevalent in the **elderly** we see.

VERTIGO/MOTION SICKNESS

MECLIZINE (Antivert)
"MECK-luh-zeen" (ANT-e-vert)
Antivert is an **anti-vertigo** drug to help get rid of the dizzy bug.

SCOPOLAMINE (Transderm-Scop)
"sco-POL-uh-mean" (trans-DERM SCOPE)
Transderm-Scop is a **trans**dermal form of **scop**olamine, for motion sickness on Caribbean cruising.

MUSCLE RELAXATION

CYCLOBENZAPRINE (Flexeril)
"sigh-clo-BENDS-uh-preen" (FLEX-er-ill)
Flexeril a muscle relaxer that improves **flexibility**.

CARISOPRODOL (Soma)
"Kar-is-uh-PRO-doll" "SEW-muh"
Soma is a muscle relaxant; it helps if you threw your back out.

VI. LOCAL ANESTHETICS

There are two major classes of local anesthetics, the esters and the amides. These are named after a molecule in the middle of their chemical structure.

Esters, such as **benzocaine (Anbesol)** are generally found only as topical agents because as an injection they are allergenic (cause allergic reactions).

Amides are much safer and **lidocaine (Xylocaine)** is considered the "gold standard". It has been used safely in pregnancy.

LOCAL ANESTHETICS – ESTER

BENZOCAINE (Anbesol)
"BENZ-oh-cane" (ANN-buh-sawl)
Anbesol hits the spot, when your tooth is aching from some rot.

LOCAL ANESTHETICS – AMIDE

LIDOCAINE (Xylocaine)
"lie-DOE-cane" (ZIE-low-cane)
Xylocaine is lid**ocaine**, often used to numb and stop pain, can be a patch or injected the same.

NERVOUS SYSTEM DRUG QUIZ (LEVEL 1)

Classify these drugs by placing the corresponding drug class letter next to each medication:

1. Alprazolam (Xanax)
2. Amitryptiline (Elavil)
3. Atomoxetine (Strattera)
4. Citalopram (Celexa)
5. Dexmethylphenidate (Focalin)
6. Divalproex (Depakote)
7. Haloperidol (Haldol)
8. Isocarboxazid (Marplan)
9. Levodopa/carbidopa (Sinemet)
10. Zolpidem (Ambien)

Nervous System Drug Classes:

A. ADHD drug/non-stimulant
B. ADHD drug/stimulant
C. Antidepressant: MAOI
D. Antidepressant: SNRI
E. Antidepressant: SSRI
F. Antidepressant: TCA
G. Antiepileptic: Newer
H. Antiepileptic: Traditional
I. Antipsychotic: Atypical
J. Antipsychotic: Typical
K. Benzodiazepine
L. Parkinson's
M. Sedative-hypnotic
N. Simple salt

Classify these drugs by placing the corresponding drug class letter next to each medication:

1. Venlafaxine
2. Diazepam
3. Phenytoin
4. Quetiapine
5. Phenelzine
6. Eszopiclone
7. Fluoxetine
8. Citalopram
9. Selegeline
10. Lithium

Nervous System Drug Classes:

A. ADHD drug/non-stimulant
B. ADHD drug/stimulant
C. Antidepressant: MAOI
D. Antidepressant: SNRI
E. Antidepressant: SSRI
F. Antidepressant: TCA
G. Antiepileptic: Newer
H. Antiepileptic: Traditional
I. Antipsychotic: Atypical
J. Antipsychotic: Typical
K. Benzodiazepine
L. Parkinson's
M. Sedative-hypnotic
N. Simple salt

CHAPTER 6 CARDIOLOGY

I. THE FOUR CLASSES OF DIURETICS

There are four generally accepted classes of diuretic:

Osmotic – These increase the osmolarity of blood and can be used to reduce intracranial pressure. An example is **mannitol (Osmitrol).**

Loop – These diuretics are named after the part of the nephron that the drug works in, the Loop of Henle, and produce significant diuresis. An example is **furosemide (Lasix).**

Thiazide – These are named after the suffix of the generic drug name such as **hydrochlorothiazide (Hydrodiuril)**. They don't produce as much diuresis as loop diuretics, but are excellent for hypertension.

Potassium sparing – These drugs will keep potassium in the body as loop and thiazide diuretics cause potassium excretion. They do not produce much diuresis. An example is **spironolactone (Aldactone).**

DIURETICS – OSMOTIC
MANNITOL (Osmitrol)
"MAN-eh-tall" (OZ-meh-trawl)
Osmitrol is an **osm**otic diuretic that helps if your brain is swellin'.

DIURETICS – LOOP
FUROSEMIDE (Lasix)
"Fyoor-OH-seh-mide" (LAY-six)
Lasix is a loop diuretic that **lasts six** hours.

DIURETICS – THIAZIDE
HYDROCHLOROTHIAZIDE (Hydrodiuril)
"High-droe-klor-oh-THIGH-uh-zide" (high-droe-DIE-yer-ill)
Hydrodiuril is combined from **diuretic** and **hydro**chlorothiazide.

DIURETICS – POTASSIUM SPARING PLUS THIAZIDE

TRIAMTERENE/HYDROCHLOROTHIAZIDE (Dyazide)
"TRY-am-terr-een/High-droe-klor-oh-THIGH-uh-zide"
(DIE-uh-zyde)
Dyazide is **dy**renium + a thi**azide** diuretic so potassium you'll keep, but still hypertension will correct.

DIURETICS – POTASSIUM SPARING

SPIRONOLACTONE (Aldactone)
"spur-oh-no-LACK-tone" (Al-DAK-tone)
Aldactone is potassium sparing and can cause gynecomastic pairing.

II. UNDERSTANDING THE ALPHAS AND BETAS

Confusion about alpha and beta adrenergic blockers (antagonists) comes from seeing receptor names (alpha and beta), instead of seeing therapeutic classes (blood pressure pills).

Let's first break down the full term. The alpha and beta are the first two letters of the Greek alphabet and are used to name the receptor. Adrenergic means works like adrenaline, so an adrenergic agonist works *like* adrenaline and an adrenergic antagonist works in the *opposite* way.

The prefix adren- refers to it being discovered in the adrenal glands. The adrenal glands are **above** (ad-) the **kidneys** (-renal) and secrete adrenaline. The suffix –ergic refers to the Greek for "works like." So these drugs work like adrenaline. Note: Adrenaline and epinephrine are the same. Epinephrine uses the Greek translation of **above** (epi-) and **kidney** (neph) to make epinephrine instead of the Latin form adrenaline.

Instead of calling **metoprolol** (**Lopressor**) an antihypertensive (a therapeutic class), it is called a beta blocker because metoprolol can also be used for migraine prevention. Instead of calling **doxazosin** (**Cardura**) an antihypertensive, it is called an alpha blocker because doxazosin can also be used for benign prostatic hyperplasia. With multiple uses we can't pin down one therapeutic class, so the receptor name alpha or beta is preferred.

There are receptor sub-types. Beta-1 receptors are in the heart (and we have one heart) and beta-2 receptors are in the lungs (and we have two lungs).

If a beta blocker is not selective, such as **propranolol (Inderal)**, for beta-1 receptors on the heart only, and blocks beta-2 receptors as well, then bronchoconstriction may occur.

Metoprolol (Lopressor) is usually preferred for this reason because it is selective for just the heart; it is called beta-1 selective.

Carvedilol (Coreg), a 3rd generation beta blocker is showing that it might be the best choice because it has vasodilating effects as well as cardiac effects.

ALPHA BLOCKERS FOR HYPERTENSION (–AZOSIN)
DOX<u>AZOSIN</u> (Cardura)
"Docks-AZ-oh-sin" (CAR-dur-uh)
Cardura provides **dura**ble **card**iac relief of hypertension.

BETA BLOCKERS – 1ST GENERATION – NON-BETA-SELECTIVE (–OLOL/–LOL)
PROPRANOLOL (Inderal)
"Pro-PRAN-uh-lawl" (IN-dur-all)
Inderal blocks beta receptors, but watch out, it blocks them all.

BETA BLOCKERS – 2ND GENERATION – BETA-SELECTIVE
METOP<u>ROLOL</u> (Lopressor)
"meh-TOE-pruh-lawl" (low-PRESS-or)
Lopressor lowers blood **pressure**.

BETA BLOCKERS – 3RD GENERATION – NON-BETA-SELECTIVE, VASODILATING
CARVEDI<u>LOL</u> (Coreg)
"car-VE-deh-lawl" (CO-reg)
Coreg regulates **cor**onary function.

III. The Renin-Angiotensin-Aldosterone-System Drugs

The **RAAS, renin-angiotensin-aldosterone system,** controls blood pressure. By defining a few words we can better understand how the drugs work.

Renin – The word come from **renal** for kidneys and this chemical changes angiotensinogen to angiotensin I. **Angiotensin I** – A chemical that can be converted to **angiotensin II**, which is a potent vasoconstrictor (blood vessel constrictor) which increases blood pressure when our body needs it. **Aldosterone** causes the retention of sodium and water further increasing blood pressure.

Angiotensin converting enzyme inhibitors (ACE inhibitors) such as **enalapril (Vasotec)** and **lisinopril (Zestril)** stop the body from creating this potent vasoconstrictor; thereby reducing hypertension.

ARBs, or angiotensin II receptor blockers, such as **losartan (Cozaar), olmesartan (Benicar)** and **valsartan (Diovan)** block or inhibit the connection between angiotensin II and the receptor that would cause vasoconstriction and are often used as an alternative to an ACE inhibitor when a patient has a cough as a side effect.

Here is a mnemonic that may help you remember the difference: *D'artagnan* the musketeer has to be *-sartan* with the b*ARB* of his blade, otherwise he's not be an *ACE* in *A-pril*, I'm afraid.

ACE Inhibitors (ACEI) (-pril)

ENALAPRIL (Vasotec)
"eh-NAL-uh-pril" (VA-zo-tech)
Vasotec **tec**hnically affects the **vas**culature, if you cough, you'll have to give it back.

LISINOPRIL (Zestril)
"lie-SIN-oh-pril" (ZES-tril)
Lisinopril thrills an overworked heart, blocking angiotensin II from getting a start.

ANGIOTENSIN II RECEPTOR BLOCKERS (ARBs) (-SARTAN)

LOSARTAN (Cozaar)
"low-SAR-tan" (CO-tsar)
Cozaar is a **co**ronary **an**giotensin II receptor **an**tagonist, with the letters in bit of a twist.

OLMESARTAN (Benicar)
"Ole'-meh-SAR-tan" (BEN-eh-car)
Benicar benefits your **car**diac condition, reduces your pressure, without any coughin'.

VALSARTAN (Diovan)
"val-SAR-tan" (DYE-oh-van)
Diovan has three of the letters of **v**als**a**rta**n**.

VASODILATORS – ANTIANGINAL

NITROGLYCERIN
"nigh-trow-GLI-sir-in"
Nitroglycerin converts to **nitr**ic oxide, a vasodilator your body abides.

IV. CALCIUM CHANNEL BLOCKERS

Calcium channel blockers classes include the **non-dihydropyridines** such as **diltiazem (Cardizem)** and **verapamil (Calan)** which affect the heart directly and can also be used as antidysrhythmics and dihydropyridines which do not directly affect the heart. **Amlodipine (Norvasc)** and **nifedipine (Procardia)** fall into this class. If a patient needs a calcium channel blocker to prevent uterine contractions, nifedipine (Procardia) would be the best choice because it does not suppress the mother's and fetus' heart. You can recognize these by the suffix –dipine.

CALCIUM CHANNEL BLOCKERS (CCBs) – NON-DIHYDROPYRIDINES

DILTIAZEM (Cardizem)
"dill-TIE-uh-zem" (CAR-deh-zem)
Cardizem is the **card**iac drug dil**t**i**a**ze**m**.

VERAPAMIL (Calan) "ver-APP-uh-mill" (KALE-en)
Vera and **Pam** are **il**(l)and need this calcium blocking cardiac pill
Calan is a **cal**cium cha**nn**el blocker.

CALCIUM CHANNEL BLOCKERS – DIHYDROPYRIDINES (–DIPINE)

AMLO<u>DIPINE</u> (Norvasc)
"am-LOW-duh-peen"(NOR-vasc)
Norvasc normalizes the **vas**culature.

NIFE<u>DIPINE</u> (Procardia)
"nigh-FED-eh-peen" (pro-CARD-e-uh)
Procardia promotes **cardiac** health, which is often better than
wealth.

V. ANTIHYPERLIPIDEMICS

Drugs for high cholesterol fall into a few categories including the
"statins" which are more properly called the HMG-CoA reductase
inhibitors, the fibrate derivatives, and the vitamins. Statins such as
atorvastatin (Lipitor), **rosuvastatin (Crestor)**, and **simvastatin**
(Zocor) are really misnamed because their suffix is –vastatin.
Nystatin (Mycostatin) has statin as a suffix, but is an antifungal
medication.

ANTIHYPERLIPIDEMICS – HMG-CoA REDUCTASE INHIBITOR (-VASTATIN)

ATOR<u>VASTATIN</u> (Lipitor)
"uh-TOR-va-stat-in" (LIP-eh-tore)
Lipitor is a **lip**id gladia**tor**.

ROSU<u>VASTATIN</u> (Crestor)
"Row-SUE-vuh-STAT-in" (CRES-tour)
Crestor de**cre**ases chol**ester**ol.

SIM<u>VASTATIN</u> (Zocor)
"SIM-va-stat-in" (ZO-cor)
Zocor reduces lipids moving through "**z**" **cor**onary arteries.

ANTIHYPERLIPIDEMICS – FIBRATE

FENOFIBRATE (Tricor)
"fen-oh-FIE-brate" (TRY-core)
Tricor lowers **tri**glycerides to help your **cor**onary status.

ANTIHYPERLIPIDEMICS – VITAMINS

NIACIN (Niaspan)
"NYE-uh-sin" (NYE-uh-span)
Niaspan helps reduce cholesterol well, but take an aspirin just before or red your cheeks will swell.

VI. ANTICOAGULANTS AND ANTIPLATELETS

The injectable anticoagulants **enoxaparin (Lovenox)** or **heparin** and oral anticoagulant **warfarin (Coumadin)** affect the coagulation in slower moving blood vessels like veins. This is in contrast to the antiplatelets **aspirin (Ecotrin)** and **clopidogrel (Plavix)** which affect how "sticky" platelets get in high pressure vessels such as arteries.

ANTICOAGULANT

ENOXAPARIN (Lovenox)
"e-knocks-uh-PEAR-in" (LOW-ven-ox)
Lovenox is a **low** molecular weight heparin for deep **vein** thrombosis prevention.

HEPARIN
"HEP-uh-rin" (HEP-uh-rin)
Heparin is an excellent anticoagulant by far. Its name comes from the Greek for liver –**hepar**.

WARFARIN (Coumadin)
"WAR-fa-rin" (KOO-ma-din)
Coumadin is an anti-**co**agulant so you can **fare** better with a stent **in**.

ANTIPLATELET

ASPIRIN [ASA] (Ecotrin)
"AS-per-in" (ECK-oh-trin)
Ecotrin is **e**nteric **co**ated aspi**rin**, keeps platelets from stickin'.

CLOPIDOGREL (Plavix)
"klo-PID-oh-grel" (PLA-vix)
Plavix vexes platelets and keeps the blood thin.

VII. CARDIAC GLYCOSIDE

A cardiac glycoside such as **digoxin (Lanoxin)** increases the force of contraction of the heart (positive inotrope) and is an antidysrhythmic which changes the electrochemistry of the heart as well. Its name comes from the digitalis plant.

CARDIAC GLYCOSIDE – POSITIVE INOTROPE -

ANTIDYSRHYTHMIC

DIGOXIN (Lanoxin)
"di-JOCKS-in" (la-KNOCKS-in)
Lanoxin uses the suffix from dig**oxin,** to keep your heartbeat rockin'.

VIII. CARDIODE TO JOY

Cardiode to Joy is a mnemonic that you can sing, hum or just say that attaches many of the common cardio drug endings and classes to their function to Beethoven's *Ode to Joy*

---

o-l-o-l-p-r-i-l-and-s-a-r-t-a-n

be-ta-block-er-ace-in-hib-i-tor-and-ARBs-suff-ix-end

as-pir-in-and-clo-pid-o-grel-both-block-plate-lets-round-a-stent

war-fa-rin-and-hep-a-rin-are-both-an-ti-co-ag-u-lants

stat-ins-low-er-chol-est-ter-ol
dig-keeps-your-heart-from-fail-in
ver-a-pa-mil-and-am-lo-di-pine
both-block-cal-cium-chan-nels.

CARDIOVASCULAR DRUG QUIZ (LEVEL 1)

Classify these drugs by placing the corresponding drug class letter next to each medication:

1. Atorvastatin (Lipitor)
2. Clopidogrel (Plavix)
3. Enalapril (Vasotec)
4. Enoxaparin (Lovenox)
5. Furosemide (Lasix)
6. Hydrochlorothiazide (Hydrodiuril)
7. Losartan (Cozaar)
8. Metoprolol (Lopressor)
9. Nifedipine (Procardia)
10. Spironolactone (Aldactone)

Cardiovascular drug classes:

A. ACE inhibitor (ACEI)
B. Alpha blocker
C. Angiotensin receptor blocker (ARB)
D. Anticoagulant
E. Antiplatelet
F. Beta blocker: selective
G. Beta blocker: non-selective
H. Calcium channel blocker (CCB) – dihydropyridine
I. Calcium channel blocker (CCB) – non-dihydropyridine
J. Cardiac glycoside
K. Diuretic: Loop
L. Diuretic: Osmotic
M. Diuretic: Potassium sparing
N. Diuretic: Thiazide
O. HMG Co-A reductase inhibitor
P. Vasodilator

CARDIOVASCULAR DRUG QUIZ (LEVEL 2)

Classify these drugs by placing the corresponding drug class letter next to each medication:

1. Diltiazem
2. Carvedilol
3. Olmesartan
4. HCTZ
5. Doxazosin
6. Amlodipine
7. Nitroglycerin
8. Lisinopril
9. Digoxin
10. Warfarin

Cardiovascular drug classes:

A. ACE inhibitor (ACEI)
B. Alpha blocker
C. Angiotensin receptor blocker (ARB)
D. Anticoagulant
E. Antiplatelet
F. Beta blocker: selective
G. Beta blocker: non-selective
H. Calcium channel blocker (CCB) – dihydropyridine
I. Calcium channel blocker (CCB) – non-dihydropyridine
J. Cardiac glycoside
K. Diuretic: Loop
L. Diuretic: Osmotic
M. Diuretic: Potassium sparing
N. Diuretic: Thiazide
O. HMG Co-A reductase inhibitor
P. Vasodilator

CHAPTER 7 ENDOCRINE

I. DIABETES AND INSULIN

Diabetes mellitus is an excess of blood sugar. There are three types: type I which is sometimes referred to as juvenile onset diabetes, type II, which can be referred to as adult-onset diabetes and gestational, a condition where pregnant women become diabetic. Depending on the condition, there are different drugs that can help lower blood sugar. Almost all oral medications have gl (for glucose) in the name. These drugs include **glipizide (Glucotrol), glyburide (DiaBeta), metformin (Glucophage)** and **rosiglitazone (Avandia)**.

Insulin for diabetes comes from the Latin word insula, which means island. The islets of Langerhans in your body have cells to produce insulin (beta cells) and cells to tell the body to raise blood glucose levels with glucagon (alpha cells).

There are four major classes of insulin used in treatment: *rapid acting* which starts working in about 15 minutes and lasts about 4 hours like **insulin lispro (Humalog)**; *slower acting* works in about 30 minutes and lasts about 6 to 8 hours like **regular insulin (Humulin R)**; *intermediate duration* like **NPH insulin (Humulin N)** which starts working in an hour or two and lasts one-half to most of the day; and *long duration* **insulin glargine (Lantus)** which starts working in about an hour and lasts 24 hours.

ANTI-DIABETIC

GLIPIZIDE (Glucotrol)
"GLIP-eh-zide" (GLUE-co-trawl)
Glucotrol controls blood **glucose** in diabetics.

GLYBURIDE (DiaBeta)
"gly-byou-ride" (die-uh-BAY-ta)
DiaBeta is for **dia**betics, working on the **beta** cells, from which insulin is let out.

METFORMIN (Glucophage)
"met-FOUR-men" (GLUE-co-fage)
Glucophage eats, or phages **glucose**, if you **met four men** on glucophage, they are diabetic.

ROSIGLITAZONE (Avandia)
"rose-eh-GLIT-uh-zone" (uh-van-DEE-uh)
Avandia is an **advan**ced **dia**betic drug.

DIABETES – RAISES BLOOD SUGAR LEVELS

GLUCAGON (GlucaGen)
"GLUE-ca-gone" (glue-ca-JEN)
Glucagen generates **gluc**ose when a patient is hypoglycemic. Use it when the glucose is gone.

INSULIN

INSULIN R (Humulin R)
"IN-su-lin" (HUE-myou-lin)
Humulin is **hum**an in**sulin**.

INSULIN GLARGINE (Lantus)
"IN-su-lin GLAR-Jean" (LAN-tuss)
Lantus lasts all day long, but take it at night, and your life will be prolonged.

II. THYROID HORMONES

Thyroid hormone (1) stimulates the heart (2) stimulates metabolism and (3) helps with growth. A hyperthyroid patient's body is using energy too quickly and needs a medication such as **propylthiouracil (PTU)** to reduce the effects of thyroid hormone. Hypothyroid patients need extra thyroid hormone, such as **levothyroxine (Synthroid)** to replace what they are missing.

DRUGS FOR HYPOTHYROIDISM

LEVOTHYROXINE (Synthroid)
"Lee-vo-thigh-ROCKS-een" (SIN-throyd)
Synthroid is a **synth**etic thy**roid** replacement, once in the morning, with no food you take it.

DRUGS FOR HYPERTHYROIDISM

PROPYLTHIOURACIL (PTU)

"PRO-pill-thigh-oh-your-uh-sill" (PEEA-tee-you)

PTU is the acronym for propylthiouracil, a thyroid hormone blocking pill.

ENDOCRINE DRUG QUIZ (LEVEL 1)

Classify these drugs by placing the corresponding drug class letter next to each medication:

1. Glipizide (Glucotrol)
2. Glucagon (GlucaGen)
3. Glyburide (DiaBeta)
4. Insulin glargine (Lantus)
5. Levothyroxine (Synthroid)
6. Metformin (Glucophage)
7. Propylthiouracil (PTU)
8. Regular insulin (Humulin R)
9. Rosiglitazone (Avandia)

Endocrine system drug classes:
   A. Anti-diabetic
   B. Long duration insulin
   C. Slower acting insulin
   D. For hypoglycemia
   E. For hypothyroidism
   F. For hyperthyroidism

ENDOCRINE DRUG QUIZ (LEVEL 2)

Classify these drugs by placing the corresponding drug class letter next to each medication:

1. Levothyroxine
2. Glucagon
3. Propylthiouracil
4. Regular insulin
5. Glipizide
6. Glyburide
7. Insulin glargine
8. Rosiglitazone
9. Metformin

Endocrine system drug classes:
A. Anti-diabetic
B. Long duration insulin
C. Slower acting insulin
D. For hypoglycemia
E. For hypothyroidism
F. For hyperthyroidism

CHAPTER 8 RENAL/REPRODUCTIVE

I. INCONTINENCE, IMPOTENCE, URINARY RETENTION, BPH

Frequently the words incontinence, impotence, urinary retention and benign prostatic hyperplasia are confused:

- **Incontinence** is the inability to retain urine.
- **Urinary retention** is a difficulty in urination.
- **Impotence** is the inability to maintain an erection.

BPH is an acronym for *benign prostatic hyperplasia* which is a non-cancerous growth of the prostate. Alpha blockers can be used for hypertension, but they also make effective drugs for BPH.

INCONTINENCE

OXYBUTYNIN (Ditropan)
"ox-e-BYOU-tin-in" (DIH-trow-pan)
Ditropan ropes and shuts down the **detrusor** muscle.

TOLTERODINE (Detrol)
"toll-TER-oh-dean" (deh-TRAWL)
Detrol helps **control** the **detrusor** muscle, keeping urine in.

URINARY RETENTION

BETHANECHOL (Urecholine)
"beth-ANN-uh-call" (your-eh-CO-lean)
Urecholine controls **ur**ine through anti**choline**rgic effects.

IMPOTENCE (PED5 INHIBITORS)—(-DENAFIL/-ALAFIL)

SIL<u>DEN</u>AFIL (Viagra)
"sill-DEN-uh-fill" (vie-AG-rah)
Viagra brings **vi**able **gr**owth.

TAD<u>AL</u>AFIL (Cialis)
"ta-DA-la-fill" (see-AL-is)
Cialis lasts the weekend.

BPH – *ALPHA BLOCKER (-AZOSIN)*

TAMSULOSIN (Flomax)
"tam-SUE-low-sin" (FLOW-Max)
Flomax allows for **max**imum urinary **flow**.

BPH – *5-ALPHA-REDUCTASE INHIBITOR (-ASTERIDE)*

DUTASTERIDE (Avodart)
"Due-TAS-ter-ide" (AH-vo-dart)
Avodart is for a prostate that's enlarged.

FINASTERIDE (Proscar)
"fin-AS-ter-ide" (pro-SCAR)
Proscar is for **pros**tate **car**e, but pregnant women should beware.

II. CONTRACEPTION

Pharmaceutical birth control traditionally came from a combined oral contraceptive pill (COCP) that has a combination of an estrogen and a progestin. Two novel delivery methods include a vaginally inserted ring **(Nuvaring)** and a transdermal patch **(OrthoEvra)**.

There are many variations of the pill including **Loestrin 24 Fe** which provides shorter menstrual periods with an iron (Fe) supplement. The tri-phasic medications such as **Tri-Sprintec** have three different doses.

CONTRACEPTION – *RING*

ETONOGESTREL/ETHINYL ESTRADIOL (NuvaRing)
"Et-oh-no-JESS-trel/ETH-in-ill Es-tra-DYE-all"(NEW-va-ring)
NuvaRing is one way to keep the stork away.

CONTRACEPTION – *PATCH*

NORELGESTROMIN/ETHINYL ESTRADIOL (OrthoEvra)
"Nor-el-JESS-tro-min/ ETH-in-ill Es-tra-DYE-all"(OR-thoe EV-rah)
OrthoEvra is a patch, put it on your arm, your abs, your buttock or back, and then take it off a week after that.

NORETHINDRONE/ETHINYL ESTRADIOL (Loestrin 24 Fe)
"Nor-ETH-in-drone/ETH-in-ill Es-tra-DYE-all" (Low-ES-trin EF-e)
Loestrin 24 Fe reduces the length of menstruation, with a little bit of iron, to keep you from an anemic condition.

NORGESTIMATE/ETHINYL ESTRADIOL (Tri-Sprintec)
"Nor-JESS-Tim-ate/ETH-in-ill Es-tra-DYE-all"
Tri-sprintec is **triphasic**, three different doses, in seven day spaces.

REPRODUCTIVE/RENAL DRUG QUIZ (LEVEL 1)

Classify these drugs by placing the corresponding drug class letter next to each medication:

1. Bethanechol (Urecholine)
2. Etonogestrel/ethinyl estradiol (NuvaRing)
3. Finasteride (Proscar)
4. Norgestimate/ethinyl estradiol (Tri-Sprintec)
5. Oxybutynin (Ditropan)
6. Sildenafil (Viagra)
7. Tadalafil (Cialis)
8. Dutasteride (Avodart)
9. Tamsulosin (Flomax)
10. Tolterodine (Detrol)

Reproductive and renal system drug classes:

A. BPH - 5-alpha-reductase inhibitor
B. BPH - alpha blocker
C. Contraception – COCP triphasic
D. Contraception – COCP with iron
E. Contraception – patch
F. Contraception – ring
G. Impotence
H. Incontinence
I. Urinary retention

REPRODUCTIVE/RENAL DRUG QUIZ (LEVEL 2)

Classify these drugs by placing the corresponding drug class letter next to each medication:

1. Dutasteride
2. Tamsulosin
3. Tolterodine
4. Tadalafil
5. Norethindrone/ethinyl estradiol Fe
6. Norelgestromin/ethinyl estradiol
7. Oxybutynin
8. Bethanechol
9. Sildenafil
10. Finasteride

Reproductive and renal system drug classes:

A. BPH - 5-alpha-reductase inhibitor
B. BPH - alpha blocker
C. Contraception – COCP triphasic
D. Contraception – COCP with iron
E. Contraception – patch
F. Contraception – ring
G. Impotence
H. Incontinence
I. Urinary retention

FINAL EXAMS

Congratulations!

You've made it through the whole book. Hopefully, you've started to commit the mnemonics to memory and found suffixes and prefixes you can count on to help you remember drug classes.

The following pages include two final exams. The first final exam provides generic and brand names for the medications and is a little easier. The second final exam only provides generic names for a greater challenge.

If you feel you want more of a review, you can take a look at the prefixes and suffixes summary in the index, then move on to the exams.

Good luck.

Best,

Dr. Guerra

Final exam 1. Questions 1-25. Chapters 1-3. (Level 1)

___1 Diphenoxylate/atropine (Lomotil)
___2 Acetaminophen (Tylenol)
___3 Allopurinol (Zyloprim)
___4 APAP/Codeine (Tylenol/Codeine)
___5 Budesonide/Formoterol (Symbicort)
___6 Colchicine (Colcrys)
___7 Esomeprazole (Nexium)
___8 Febuxostat (Uloric)
___9 Guaifenesin/DM (Robitussin DM)
__10 Fluticasone/Salmeterol (Advair)
__11 Hydrocodone/APAP (Vicodin)
__12 Fentanyl (Duragesic)
__13 Famotidine (Pepcid)
__14 Docusate (Colace)
__15 Celecoxib (Celebrex)
__16 Aspirin [ASA] (Ecotrin)
__17 Alendronate (Fosamax)
__18 Albuterol (ProAir)
__19 ASA/APAP/Caffeine (Excedrin)
__20 Bismuth (Pepto-Bismol)
__21 Calcium Carbonate (Tums)
__22 Guaifenesin/codeine (Cheratussin AC)
__23 Cetirizine (Zyrtec)
__24 Diphenhydramine (Benadryl)
__25 Etanercept (Enbrel)

a. 1st generation antihistamine
b. 2nd generation antihistamine
c. 5-HT receptor antagonist
d. Antacid
e. Anticholinergic for asthma
f. Anti-diarrheal
g. Anti-gout
h. Anti-nausea
i. Bisphosphonate
j. DMARD
k. H_2 blocker
l. Laxative
m. Mucolytic/cough
n. Non-narcotic analgesic combo
o. Non-narcotic analgesic
p. NSAID
q. Opioid analgesic
r. Proton pump inhibitor
s. Short-acting bronchodilator
t. Steroid/bronchodilator

Final exam 1. Questions 26-50. Chapter 4. (Level 1)

__26 Zidovudine (Retrovir)
__27 Amoxicillin/clavulanate (Augmentin)
__28 Ceftriaxone (Rocephin)
__29 Doxycycline (Doryx)
__30 Levofloxacin (Levaquin)
__31 SMZ/TMP (Bactrim)
__32 Cephalexin (Keflex)
__33 Ethambutol (Myambutol)
__34 Rifampin (Rifadin)
__35 Isoniazid (INH)
__36 Amikacin (Amikin)
__37 Cefepime (Maxipime)
__38 Amphotericin B (Fungizone)
__39 Amoxicillin (Amoxil)
__40 Azithromycin (Zithromax)
__41 Fluconazole (Diflucan)
__42 Oseltamivir (Tamiflu)
__43 Tetracycline (Sumycin)
__44 Clarithromycin (Biaxin)
__45 Gentamicin (Garamycin)
__46 Pyrazinamide (PZA)
__47 Nystatin (Mycostatin)
__48 Erythromycin (E-Mycin)
__49 Ciprofloxacin (Cipro)
__50 Acyclovir (Zovirax)

a. 1st generation cephalosporin
b. 2nd generation cephalosporin
c. 3rd generation cephalosporin
d. 4th generation cephalosporin
e. Antibiotic: aminoglycoside
f. Antibiotic: fluoroquinolone
g. Antibiotic: macrolide
h. Antibiotic: penicillin
i. Antibiotic: sulfa
j. Antibiotic: tetracycline
k. Antifungal
l. Antituberculosis
m. Antiviral: herpes
n. Antiviral: HIV
o. Antiviral: Influenza

Final exam 1. Questions 51-75. Chapter 5. (Level 1)

__51 Carisoprodol (Soma)
__52 Carbamazepine (Tegretol)
__53 Cyclobenzaprine (Flexeril)
__54 Divalproex (Depakote)
__55 Gabapentin (Neurontin)
__56 Lithium
__57 Meclizine (Antivert)
__58 Lidocaine (Lidoderm)
__59 Fluoxetine (Prozac)
__60 Diazepam (Valium)
__61 Clonazepam (Klonopin)
__62 Benzocaine (Anbesol)
__63 Amitriptyline (Elavil)
__64 Atomoxetine (Strattera)
__65 Dexmethylphenidate (Focalin)
__66 Escitalopram (Lexapro)
__67 Haloperidol (Haldol)
__68 Lorazepam (Ativan)
__69 Levodopa/carbidopa (Sinemet)
__70 Donepezil (Aricept)
__71 Citalopram (Celexa)
__72 Alprazolam (Xanax)
__73 Chlorpromazine (Thorazine)
__74 Eszopiclone (Lunesta)
__75 Isocarboxazid (Marplan)

a. ADHD drug/non-stimulant
b. ADHD drug/stimulant
c. Alzheimer's
d. Antidepressant: MAOI
e. Antidepressant: SNRI
f. Antidepressant: SSRI
g. Antidepressant: TCA
h. Antiepileptic: newer
i. Antiepileptic: traditional
j. Antiepileptic: atypical
k. Antipsychotic: typical
l. Benzodiazepine
m. Local anesthetic
n. Muscle relaxer
o. Parkinson's
p. Sedative-hypnotic
q. Simple salt
r. Vertigo/motion sickness

Final exam 1. Questions 76-100. Chapters 6-8. (Level 1)

__76 Norethindrone/ethinyl estradiol Fe (Loestrin Fe)
__77 Bethanechol (Urecholine)
__78 Amlodipine (Norvasc)
__79 Diltiazem (Cardizem)
__80 Glucagon (GlucaGen)
__81 Finasteride (Proscar)
__82 Hydrochlorothiazide (Hydrodiuril)
__83 Regular insulin (Insulin R)
__84 HCTZ/triamterene (Dyazide)
__85 Oxybutynin (Ditropan)
__86 Clopidogrel (Plavix)
__87 Norgestimate/ethinyl estradiol (Tri-Sprintec)
__88 Propranolol (Inderal)
__89 Furosemide (Lasix)
__90 Enalapril (Vasotec)
__91 Insulin glargine (Lantus)
__92 Enoxaparin (Lovenox)
__93 Atorvastatin (Lipitor)
__94 Digoxin (Lanoxin)
__95 Norelgestromin/ethinyl estradiol (OrthoEvra)
__96 Dutasteride (Avodart)
__97 Glipizide (Glucotrol)
__98 Heparin
__99 Glyburide (DiaBeta)
_100 Etonogestrel/ethinyl estradiol (Nuvaring)

a. ACE inhibitor
b. Angiotensin receptor blocker
c. Anticoagulant
d. Antidiabetic
e. Antiplatelet
f. Beta blocker
g. BPH: 5-alpha-reductase inhib
h. BPH: alpha blocker
i. Calcium channel blocker
j. Cardiac glycoside
k. Contraception
l. Diuretic
m. For hypoglycemia
n. For hyperthyroidism
o. For hypothyroidism
p. HMG CoA reductase inhibitor
q. Impotence
r. Incontinence
s. Longer duration insulin
t. Slower acting insulin
u. Urinary retention
v. Vasodilator

Final Exam 2. Questions 1-25. Chapters 1-3. (Level 2)

___1 Loratadine
___2 Diphenhydramine
___3 Ranitidine
___4 Pseudoephedrine
___5 Pantoprazole
___6 Naproxen
___7 Mometasone
___8 Mesalamine
___9 Loperamide
__10 Diphenoxylate/atropine
__11 Ibuprofen
__12 Magnesium hydroxide
__13 Methotrexate [MTX]
__14 Cetirizine
__15 Oxycodone
__16 Prednisone
__17 Sumatriptan
__18 Tiotropium
__19 Promethazine
__20 Polyethylene glycol
__21 Oxycodone/APAP
__22 Omeprazole
__23 Ondansetron
__24 Morphine
__25 Methylprednisolone

a. 1st generation antihistamine
b. 2nd generation antihistamine
c. 5-HT receptor antagonist
d. Antacid
e. Anticholinergic for asthma
f. Anti-diarrheal
g. Anti-gout
h. Anti-nausea
i. Decongestant
j. DMARD
k. H$_2$ blocker
l. Laxative
m. Mucolytic/cough
n. Non-narcotic analgesic combo
o. Non-narcotic analgesic
p. NSAID
q. Opioid analgesic
r. Proton pump inhibitor
s. Steroid
t. Ulcerative colitis

Final exam 2. Questions 26-50. Chapter 4. (Level 2)

__26 Doxycycline
__27 Amoxicillin
__28 SMZ/TMP
__29 Amphotericin B
__30 Erythromycin
__31 Ceftriaxone
__32 Rifampin
__33 Isoniazid
__34 Cephalexin
__35 Ethambutol
__36 Nystatin
__37 Tetracycline
__38 Valacyclovir
__39 Zanamavir
__40 Amikacin
__41 Gentamicin
__42 Clarithromycin
__43 Cefepime
__44 Oseltamivir
__45 Fluconazole
__46 Ciprofloxacin
__47 Amoxicillin/clavulanate
__48 Levofloxacin
__49 Pyrazinamide
__50 Zidovudine

a. 1st generation cephalosporin
b. 2nd generation cephalosporin
c. 3rd generation cephalosporin
d. 4th generation cephalosporin
e. Antibiotic: aminoglycoside
f. Antibiotic: fluoroquinolone
g. Antibiotic: macrolide
h. Antibiotic: penicillin
i. Antibiotic: sulfa
j. Antibiotic: tetracycline
k. Antifungal
l. Antituberculosis
m. Antiviral: herpes
n. Antiviral: HIV
o. Antiviral: influenza

Final exam 2. Questions 51-75. Chapter 5. (Level 2)

__51 Selegeline
__52 Sertraline
__53 Quetiapine
__54 Phenelzine
__55 Meclizine
__56 Isocarboxazid
__57 Gabapentin
__58 Levodopa/carbidopa
__59 Memantine
__60 Phenytoin
__61 Ramelton
__62 Tranylcypromine
__63 Venlafaxine
__64 Trazodone
__65 Pregabalin
__66 Olanzapine
__67 Lorazepam
__68 Haloperidol
__69 Lidocaine
__70 Paroxetine
__71 Risperidone
__72 Zolpidem
__73 Scopolamine
__74 Methylphenidate
__75 Lithium

a. ADHD drug/non-stimulant
c. Alzheimer's
e. Antidepressant: SNRI
g. Antidepressant: TCA
i. Antiepileptic: Traditional
k. Antipsychotic: Typical
m.Local anesthetic
o. Parkinson's
q.Simple salt

b. ADHD drug/stimulant
d. Antidepressant: MAOI
f. Antidepressant: SSRI
h. Antiepileptic: Newer
j. Antipsychotic: Atypical
l. Benzodiazepine
n. Muscle relaxer
p. Sedative-hypnotic
r. Vertigo/motion sickness

Final exam 2. Questions 76-100. Chapters 6-8. (Level 2)

__76 Levothyroxine
__77 Spironolactone
__78 Tolterodine
__79 Rosuvastatin
__80 Carvedilol
__81 Olmesartan
__82 Lovastatin
__83 Lisinopril
__84 Metformin
__85 Oxybutynin
__86 Simvastatin
__87 Valsartan
__88 Tamsulosin
__89 Nifedipine
__90 Propylthiouracil
__91 Losartan
__92 Propranolol
__93 Tadalafil
__94 Sildenafil
__95 Verapamil
__96 Rosiglitazone
__97 Enalapril
__98 Mannitol
__99 Metoprolol
_100 Warfarin

a. ACE inhibitor
c. Anticoagulant
e. Antiplatelet
g. BPH: 5-alpha-reductase inhib
i. Calcium channel blocker
k. Contraception
m. For hypoglycemia
o. For hypothyroidism
q. Impotence
s. Longer duration insulin
u. Urinary retention

b. Angiotensin receptor blocker
d. Antidiabetic
f. Beta blocker
h. BPH: alpha blocker
j. Cardiac glycoside
l. Diuretic
n. For hyperthyroidism
p. HMG CoA reductase inhibitor
r. Incontinence
t. Slower acting insulin
v. Vasodilator

APPENDIX

ANSWERS TO COMMONLY CONFUSED MEDICATIONS QUIZ

1. Aricept is an Alzheimer's medication.
   Aciphex is a proton pump inhibitor.

2. Captopril is an ACE inhibitor.
   Carvedilol is a beta blocker.

3. Celebrex is a non-steroidal anti-inflammatory drug.
   Celexa is an antidepressant.

4. Colace is a stool softener.
   Cozaar is a blood pressure medication.

5. Atorvastatin is a cholesterol-lowering medicine.
   Nystatin is an antifungal.

6. Levothyroxine is for thyroid replacement.
   Digoxin is to strengthen cardiac contraction.

7. Lopressor is a beta blocker for blood pressure.
   Lyrica is a medicine to relieve neuropathic pain.

8. Motrin is a non-steroidal anti-inflammatory drug.
   Neurontin is for neuropathic pain.

9. Oxycontin is long-acting oxycodone.
   Oxycodone is short-acting oxycodone.

10. Plavix is a blood thinner.
    Paxil is an antidepressant.

ANSWERS TO DRUG PRACTICE QUIZZES (LEVEL 1)

Gastrointestinal drugs
1. A 2. E 3. D 4. E 5. F 6. B 7. A 8. G 9. F 10. C

Musculoskeletal drugs
1. E 2.C 3. F 4. B 5. D 6. I 7. I 8. G 9. H 10. A

Respiratory drugs
1. I 2. B 3. A 4. J 5. F 6. C 7. B 8. E 9. D 10. G

Immune system drugs
1. H 2. G 3. D 4. C 5. K 6. E 7. L 8. F 9. K 10. M

Nervous system drugs
1. K 2. F 3. A 4. E 5. B 6. H 7. J 8. C 9. L 10. M

Cardiovascular system drugs
1. O 2. E 3. A 4. D 5. K 6. N 7. C 8. F 9. H 10. M

Endocrine system drugs
1. A 2. D 3. A 4. B 5. E 6. A 7. F 8. C 9. A

Renal and reproductive system drugs
1. I 2. F 3. A 4. C 5. H 6. G 7. G 8. A 9. B 10. H

ANSWERS TO DRUG PRACTICE QUIZZES (LEVEL 2)

Gastrointestinal drugs
1. B 2. B 3. F 4. D 5. C 6. A 7. E 8. D 9. B 10. E

Musculoskeletal drugs
1. D 2. I 3. I 4. G 5. B 6. C 7. B 8. G 9. C 10. I

Respiratory drugs
1. J 2. F 3. H 4. J 5. D 6. B 7. A 8. I 9. E 10. G

Immune system drugs
1. L 2. K 3. E 4. F 5. L 6. M 7. A 8. I 9. G 10. O

Nervous system drugs
1. D 2. K 3. H 4. I 5. C 6. M 7. E 8. E 9. L 10. N

Cardiovascular system drugs
1. I 2. G 3. C 4. N 5. B 6. H 7. P 8. A 9. J 10. D

Endocrine system drugs
1. E 2. D 3. F 4. C 5. A 6. A 7. B 8. A 9. A

Renal and reproductive system drugs
1. A 2. B 3. H 4. G 5. D 6. E 7. H 8. I 9. G 10. A

ANSWERS TO FINAL EXAM (LEVEL 1)

1	f	26	n	51	n	76	k
2	o	27	h	52	i	77	u
3	g	28	c	53	n	78	i
4	q	29	j	54	i	79	i
5	t	30	f	55	h	80	m
6	g	31	i	56	q	81	g
7	r	32	a	57	r	82	l
8	g	33	l	58	m	83	t
9	m	34	l	59	f	84	l
10	t	35	l	60	l	85	r
11	q	36	e	61	l	86	e
12	q	37	d	62	m	87	k
13	k	38	k	63	g	88	f
14	l	39	h	64	a	89	l
15	p	40	g	65	b	90	a
16	p	41	k	66	f	91	s
17	i	42	o	67	k	92	c
18	s	43	j	68	l	93	p
19	n	44	g	69	o	94	j
20	f	45	e	70	c	95	k
21	d	46	l	71	f	96	g

22 m	47 k	72 l	97 d
23 b	48 g	73 k	98 c
24 a	49 f	74 p	99 d
25 j	50 m	75 d	100 k

ANSWERS TO FINAL EXAM (LEVEL 2)

1 b	26 j	51 o	76 o
2 a	27 h	52 f	77 l
3 k	28 i	53 j	78 r
4 i	29 k	54 d	79 p
5 r	30 g	55 r	80 f
6 p	31 c	56 d	81 b
7 s	32 l	57 h	82 p
8 t	33 l	58 o	83 a
9 f	34 a	59 c	84 d
10 f	35 l	60 i	85 r
11 p	36 k	61 p	86 p
12 d	37 j	62 d	87 b
13 j	38 m	63 e	88 h
14 b	39 o	64 p	89 i
15 q	40 e	65 h	90 n
16 s	41 e	66 j	91 b
17 c	42 g	67 l	92 f
18 e	43 d	68 k	93 q
19 h	44 o	69 m	94 q
20 l	45 k	70 f	95 i
21 q	46 f	71 j	96 d
22 r	47 h	72 p	97 a
23 h	48 f	73 r	98 l
24 q	49 l	74 b	99 f
25 s	50 n	75 q	100 c

COMMON PREFIXES AND SUFFIXES SUMMARY

(ALPHABETICAL)

-asteride – 5-alpha-reductase inhibitors
-azole – Antifungal [-prazole will usually be a PPI]
-cillin – Penicillin antibiotic
-cycline – Tetracycline antibiotic
-denafil, -dalafil – PED5 inhibitors for erectile dysfunction
-dipine – Calcium channel blocker [some, not verapamil, diltiazem]
-dronate – Bisphosphonate for osteoporosis
-floxacin – Fluoroquinolone antibiotic
-olol, -lol – Beta blocker [avoid confusion with similar –terol]
-mab – Monoclonal antibody
-micin, mycin – Aminoglycoside antibiotic [not -thromycin]
-parin – Anticoagulant
-prazole – PPI – Acidic GI conditions [-azole alone is not enough]
-pril – Angiotensin converting enzyme inhibitor (ACEI)
-sartan – Angiotensin II receptor blocker (ARB)
-sone – Corticosteroid for inflammation
-terol – Bronchodilator for asthma [confusion with –olol, –lol]
-tidine – H_2 Blocker – acidic GI conditions
-thromycin – Macrolide antibiotic
-triptan – Serotonin receptor agonist (migraines)
-vastatin – HMG Co-A reductase inhibitors ("statins")
                    [Caution: "nystatin" is an antifungal]
-vir – Antiviral
-zosin, -osin – Alpha-blocker for BPH or hypertension
-zepam, -zolam – Benzodiazepine for anxiety, sleep
Cef-, ceph- Cephalosporin antibiotic
Sulfa- Sulfa antibiotic

(BY PHYSIOLOGIC SYSTEM)

Chapter 1 – GI
-prazole – PPI – Acidic GI conditions [Confused with -azole]
-tidine H_2 blocker – Acidic GI conditions

Chapter 2 – Musculoskeletal
-dronate – Bisphosphonate for osteoporosis
-mab – Monoclonal antibody

Chapter 3 – Respiratory
-terol – Bronchodilator for asthma [confusion with –olol, –lol]
-sone – Corticosteroid for inflammation

Chapter 4 – Immune
-azole – Antifungal [don't confuse with prazole]
-cillin – Penicillin antibiotic
-cycline – Tetracycline antibiotic
-floxacin – Fluoroquinolone antibiotic
-micin, mycin – Aminoglycoside antibiotic [not -thromycin]
-thromycin – Macrolide antibiotic
-vir – Antiviral

Sulfa- Sulfa antibiotic
Cef-, ceph- Cephalosporin antibiotic

Chapter 5 – Nervous
-triptan – Serotonin receptor agonist (migraines)
-zepam, -zolam – Benzodiazepine for anxiety, sleep

Chapter 6 – Cardiology
-dipine – Calcium channel blocker [*some* not verapamil, diltiazem)
-olol, -lol – Beta blocker [avoid confusion with –terol]
-parin – Anticoagulant
-pril – Angiotensin converting enzyme inhibitor (ACEI)
-sartan – Angiotensin II receptor blocker (ARB)
-vastatin – HMG Co-A reductase inhibitors ("statins")
-zosin, -osin – Alpha blocker for BPH or hypertension

Chapter 8 – Renal/Reproductive
-denafil, -dalafil – PED5 inhibitors for erectile dysfunction
-asteride – 5-alpha-reductase inhibitors

DRUGS BY CLASS – GENERIC (BRAND)

CHAPTER 1 – GASTROINTESTINAL

Antacids
CALCIUM CARBONATE (Tums)
MAGNESIUM HYDROXIDE (Milk of Magnesia)
H₂ blockers (-tidine)
CIMETIDINE (Tagamet)
FAMOTIDINE (Pepcid)
Proton pump inhibitors (-prazole)
ESOMEPRAZOLE (Nexium)
OMEPRAZOLE (Prilosec)
PANTOPRAZOLE (Protonix)
Anti-nausea (anti-emetics)
ONDANSETRON (Zofran)
PROMETHAZINE (Phenergan)
Anti-diarrheals
BISMUTH SUBSALICYLATE (Pepto-Bismol)
DIPHENOXYLATE/ATROPINE (Lomotil)
LOPERAMIDE (Imodium)
Constipation – Osmotic
POLYETHYLENE GLYCOL (Miralax)
Constipation – Stool softener
DOCUSATE SODIUM (Colace)
Ulcerative colitis
MESALAMINE (Asacol)

CHAPTER 2 - MUSCULOSKELETAL

Analgesics – NSAIDs – COX-1 inhibitors
ASPIRIN [ASA] (Ecotrin)
IBUPROFEN (Motrin)
NAPROXEN (Aleve)
MELOXICAM (Mobic)
Analgesics – NSAIDs – COX-2 inhibitors
CELECOXIB (Celebrex)
Analgesic – non-narcotic
ACETAMINOPHEN [APAP] (Tylenol)

Opioid analgesics – Schedule II
FENTANYL (Duragesic)
MORPHINE
OXYCODONE (OxyIR)
OXYCODONE/ACETAMINOPHEN (Endocet/Oxycontin)
Opioid analgesics - Schedule III
HYDROCODONE/ACETAMINOPHIN (Vicodin)
ACETAMINOPHEN WITH CODEINE (Tylenol with Codeine)
Opioid analgesics - Unscheduled
TRAMADOL (Ultram)
Migraine – OTC – NSAID/non-narcotic analgesic
ASPIRIN/ACETAMINOPHEN/CAFFEINE (Excedrin Migraine)
Migraine – Rx - 5-HT receptor agonist (-triptan)
SUMA<u>TRIPTAN</u> (Imitrex)
DMARDs
ETANERCEPT (Enbrel)
METHOTREXATE (Rheumatrex)
Osteoporosis – bisphosphonate (-dronate)
ALEN<u>DRONATE</u> (Fosamax)
IBAN<u>DRONATE</u> (Boniva)
Anti-Gout – for acute attacks
COLCHICINE (Cholcrys)
Anti-Gout – uric acid reducers
ALLOPURINOL (Zyloprim)
FEBUXOSTAT (Uloric)

CHAPTER 3 - RESPIRATORY

Antihistamine – 1st generation
DIPHENHYDRAMINE (Benadryl)
Antihistamine – 2nd generation
CETIRIZINE (Zyrtec)
LORATADINE (Claritin)
Mucolytic/cough suppressant - OTC
GUAIFENESIN/DEXTROMETHORPHAN (Robitussin DM)
Mucolytic/cough suppressant – Rx
GUAIFENESIN/CODEINE (Cheratussin AC)
Allergic Rhinitis – nasal steroid – (-sone)
MOMETA<u>SONE</u> (Nasonex)

Asthma – oral steroids (-sone/-lone)
METHYLPREDNISO<u>LONE</u> (Medrol)
PREDNI<u>SONE</u> (Deltasone)
Asthma – short acting beta agonist (-terol)
ALBU<u>TEROL</u> (ProAir)
Asthma – steroid/long acting bronchodilator
BUDE<u>SONIDE</u>/FORMO<u>TEROL</u> (Symbicort)
FLUTICA<u>SONE</u>/SALME<u>TEROL</u> (Advair)
Asthma/COPD – Anti-cholinergic (-tropium)
TIO<u>TROPIUM</u> (Spiriva)
Asthma – Leukotriene receptor antagonist (-lukast)
MONTELUKAST (Singulair)
Congestion – Decongestant
PSEUDOEPHEDRINE (Sudafed)
Anaphylaxis
EPINEPHRINE (EpiPen)

CHAPTER 4 – IMMUNE

Antibiotics: Penicillins
AMOXI<u>CILLIN</u> (Amoxil)
Antibiotics: Penicillin/Beta-lactamase inhibitor
AMOXI<u>CILLIN</u>/CLAVULANATE (Augmentin)
Antibiotics: Cephalosporins (cef-/ceph-)
<u>CEPH</u>ALEXIN (Keflex)
<u>CEF</u>TRIAXONE (Rocephin)
<u>CEF</u>EPIME (Maxipime)
Antibiotics: Macrolides (-thromycin)
ERY<u>THROMYCIN</u> (E-Mycin)
CLARI<u>THROMYCIN</u> (Biaxin)
AZI<u>THROMYCIN</u> (Zithromax)
Antibiotics: Fluoroquinolones (-floxacin)
CIPRO<u>FLOXACIN</u> (Cipro)
LEVO<u>FLOXACIN</u> (Levaquin)
Antibiotics: Tetracyclines (–cycline)
DOXY<u>CYCLINE</u> (Doryx)
TETRA<u>CYCLINE</u> (Sumycin)
Antibiotics: Aminoglycosides
AMIKA<u>CIN</u> (Amikin)
GENTA<u>MICIN</u> (Garamycin)

Antibiotics: Lincosamide
CLINDA<u>MYCIN</u> (Cleocin)
Antibiotic: Nitroimidazole / Anti-protozoal
METRONIDAZOLE (Flagyl)
Antibiotics: Dihidrofolate reductase inhibitor (Sulfa-)
SULFAMETHOXAZOLE/TRIMETHOPRIM (SMZ-TMP)
Antibiotics: Glycopeptide
VANCO<u>MYCIN</u> (Vancocin)
Anti-tuberculosis agents
ETHAMBUTOL (Myambutol)
ISONIAZID (INH)
PYRAZINAMIDE (PZA)
RIFAMPIN (Rifadin)
Antifungals
AMPHOTERICIN B (Fungizone)
FLUCON<u>AZOLE</u> (Diflucan)
NYSTATIN (Mycostatin)
Antivirals – Influenza (-vir)
OSELTAMI<u>VIR</u> (Tamiflu)
ZANAMI<u>VIR</u> (Relenza)
Antivirals – Herpes (-vir)
ACYCLO<u>VIR</u> (Zovirax)
VALACYCLO<u>VIR</u> (Valtrex)
Antivirals – HIV (-vir)
ZIDOVUDINE (Retrovir)

CHAPTER 5 – NERVOUS SYSTEM

Sedative-hypnotics (sleeping pills)
ESZOPICLONE (Lunesta)
RAMELTON (Rozerem)
TRAZODONE (Desyrel)
ZOLPIDEM (Ambien)
Selective serotonin reuptake inhibitors (SSRIs)
CITALOPRAM (Celexa)
ESCITALOPRAM (Lexapro)
FLUOXETINE (Prozac)
PAROXETINE (Paxil)
SERTRALINE (Zoloft)

Serotonin-Norepinephrine reuptake inhibitors (SNRIs)
VENLAFAXINE (Effexor)
Tricyclic antidepressants (TCAs)
AMITRIPTYLINE (Elavil)
Monoamine oxidase inhibitors (MAOIs)
ISOCARBOXAZID (Marplan)
PHENELZINE (Nardil)
TRANYLCYPROMINE (Parnate)
Benzodiazepines (-zolam/–zepam)
ALPRAZOLAM (Xanax)
CLONAZEPAM (Klonopin)
DIAZEPAM (Valium)
LORAZEPAM (Ativan)
ADHD medications – stimulant – Schedule II
DEXMETHYLPHENIDATE (Focalin)
METHYLPHENIDATE (Concerta)
ADHD medications – non-stimulant – non-scheduled
ATOMOXETINE (Strattera)
Bipolar Disorder – Simple salt
LITHIUM
Schizophrenia – (typical antipsychotic/low potency)
CHLORPROMAZINE (Thorazine)
Schizophrenia – (typical antipsychotic/high potency)
HALOPERIDOL (Haldol)
Schizophrenia – (atypical antipsychotic)
OLANZAPINE (Zyprexa)
QUETIAPINE (Seroquel)
RISPERIDONE (Risperdal)
Antiepileptics – traditional
CARBAMAZEPINE (Tegretol)
DIVALPROEX (Depakote)
PHENYTOIN (Dilantin)
Antiepileptics – newer
GABAPENTIN (Neurontin)
PREGABALIN (Lyrica)
Drugs for Alzheimer's
DONEPEZIL (Aricept)
MEMANTINE (Namenda)

Drugs for Parkinson's
LEVODOPA/CARBIDOPA (Sinemet)
SELEGILINE (Eldepryl)
Vertigo/motion sickness
MECLIZINE (Antivert)
SCOPOLAMINE (Transderm-Scop)
Muscle relaxation
CYCLOBENZAPRINE (Flexeril)
CARISOPRODOL (Soma)
Local Anesthetics – Ester
BENZOCAINE (Anbesol)
Local Anesthetics – Amide
LIDOCAINE (Xylocaine)

CHAPTER 6 – CARDIOLOGY

Diuretics
MANNITOL (Osmitrol)
FUROSEMIDE (Lasix)
HYDROCHLOROTHIAZIDE (Hydrodiuril)
TRIAMTERENE/HYDROCHLOROTHIAZIDE (Dyazide)
SPIRONOLACTONE (Aldactone)
Alpha blockers (for hypertension) (–azosin)
DOXAZOSIN (Cardura)
Beta blockers – 1st generation – non-beta selective (–olol/–lol)
PROPRANOLOL (Inderal)
Beta blockers – 2nd generation – beta selective
METOPROLOL (Lopressor)
Beta blockers – 3rd generation – non-beta selective, vasodilating
CARVEDILOL (Coreg)
ACE Inhibitors (ACEI) – have the suffix -pril
ENALAPRIL (Vasotec)
LISINOPRIL (Zestril)
Angiotensin II receptor blockers (ARBs) – have the suffix sartan
LOSARTAN (Cozaar)
OLMESARTAN (Benicar)
VALSARTAN (Diovan)
Vasodilators – antianginal
NITROGLYCERIN

Calcium channel blockers (CCBs) – Non-dihydropyridines
DILTIAZEM (Cardizem)
VERAPAMIL (Calan)
Calcium channel blockers – Dihydropyridines (–dipine)
AMLODIPINE (Norvasc)
NIFEDIPINE (Procardia)
Antihyperlipidemics (HMG-CoA reductase inhibitor) (-vastatin)
ATORVASTATIN (Lipitor)
ROSUVASTATIN (Crestor)
SIMVASTATIN (Zocor)
Antihyperlipidemics – fibrate
FENOFIBRATE (Tricor)
Antihyperlipidemics – vitamins
NIACIN (Niaspan)
Anticoagulant
ENOXAPARIN (Lovenox)
HEPARIN
WARFARIN (Coumadin)
Antiplatelet
ASPIRIN [ASA] (Ecotrin)
CLOPIDOGREL (Plavix)
Cardiac glycoside – positive inotrope/antidysrhythmic
DIGOXIN (Lanoxin)

CHAPTER 7 - ENDOCRINE

Anti-diabetic
GLIPIZIDE (Glucotrol)
GLYBURIDE (DiaBeta)
METFORMIN (Glucophage)
ROSIGLITAZONE (Avandia)
Hypoglycemia
GLUCAGON (GlucaGen)
Insulin
INSULIN R (Humulin R)
INSULIN GLARGINE (Lantus)
Drugs for hypothyroidism
LEVOTHYROXINE (Synthroid)
Drugs for hyperthyroidism
PROPYLTHIOURACIL (PTU)

CHAPTER 8 – RENAL/REPRODUCTIVE

Incontinence
OXYBUTYNIN (Ditropan)
TOLTERODINE (Detrol)
Urinary retention
BETHANECHOL (Urecholine)
Impotence (PED5 inhibitors) (-denafil/-alafil)
SILDENAFIL (Viagra)
TADALAFIL (Cialis)
BPH – alpha blocker (-azosin)
TAMSULOSIN (Flomax)
BPH – 5-alpha-reducase inhibitor (-asteride)
DUTASTERIDE (Avodart)
FINASTERIDE (Proscar)
Contraception – ring
ETONOGESTREL/ETHINYL ESTRADIOL (NuvaRing)
Contraception – patch
NORELGESTROMIN/ETHINYL ESTRADIOL (OrthoEvra)
Contraception – combined oral contraceptive pill (COCP)
NORETHINDRONE/ETHINYL ESTRADIOL (Loestrin 24 Fe)
NORGESTIMATE/ETHINYL ESTRADIOL (Tri-Sprintec)

ACKNOWLEDGEMENTS

To Mindy, Brielle, Rianne, and Teagan

Special thanks to Marc Dickinson M.F.A. at Des Moines Area Community College and Dr. Steve Pett at Iowa State University for helping me articulate my thoughts as a parent, pharmacist, and teacher through their writing classes.

My students below who contributed parts or all of certain drug mnemonics and Stephanie Bruner for her editorial work.

Andrea Corns, Toradol
Felisha Montero, -sartan/-pril
Ginger Cochran, Marplan
Karin Hanson, verapamil, methotrexate
Kristine Newton, -sartan/–pril, -olol, beta blockers, alprazolam
Mickenzie Block, spironolactone
Samantha Studer, isocarboxazid
Tracy Thompson, lisinopril

ABOUT THE AUTHOR

Tony Guerra graduated with his Doctor of Pharmacy from the University of Maryland in Baltimore, Maryland and his Bachelor of Arts in English from Iowa State University and has been a practicing pharmacist for 15 years. He lives in Ankeny, Iowa, with his wife Mindy and triplet daughters Brielle, Rianne, and Teagan. He teaches at Des Moines Area Community College as a chair and instructor of the pharmacy technician program and also teaches health science anatomy, organic chemistry, and biochemistry. His writing has been featured in "Expressions" and "Sketch" student literary magazines. He has also written: Prepharmacy: Getting into Pharmacy School without Drowning in Debt

Notes:

Made in the USA
San Bernardino, CA
01 March 2014